Get Back in the Game

Get Back in the Game

OVERCOMING the EIGHT OBSTACLES to OPTIMAL FEMALE HEALTH and PERFORMANCE

JACKIE CRUICKSHANK COHEN
M.A. PN, PHC, ph 360

Get Back in the Game: Overcoming the Eight Obstacles to Optimal Female Health and Performance

Copyright © 2020 by PRX Press.

All rights reserved. No part of this publication may be reproduced, distributed, or transmitted in any form or by any means, including photocopying, recording, or other electronic or mechanical methods, without the prior written permission of the publisher, except in the case of brief quotations embodied in critical reviews and certain other noncommercial uses permitted by copyright law.

www.performanceprescription.com

Printed in the United States of America

ISBN-13:

First Edition

Cover and interior design: Adina Cucicov

Table of Contents

An Introduction		vii
Obstacle One	An Energy Imbalance	1
Obstacle Two	Macronutrient Imbalances	41
Obstacle Three	Poor Cellular Health	73
Obstacle Four	Digestive Dysfunction	117
Obstacle Five	An Imbalanced Nervous System	155
Obstacle Six	Hormonal Imbalances	191
Obstacle Seven	Toxic Overload	229
Obstacle Eight	The Lack of Objective Feedback and Guidance	279
Conclusion		309
Appendix One	Making Sustainable Food Choices	313
Appendix Two	Building a Better Food Pyramid	315
Appendix Three	Using Targeted Nutritional Supplements	325
Appendix Four	The Abbreviated Guide to Identifying and Minimizing Toxins	329
Appendix Five	Resources	337

Many thanks to Eirann Cohen, Wilma Schwarz Egg, and Amy Bassett Williams—my team of impeccable proofreaders.

To Ethan and Rick Cohen for their optimism and ongoing support.

And to Dr. Robert Brown, who taught me how to write.

An Introduction

Women are different than men. They differ in height, weight, muscle mass, body composition, and aerobic capacity. They also differ in terms of their predisposition to both illness and injury.

When compared to their male counterparts, women are four times more likely to develop chronic fatigue, three times more likely to develop an autoimmune disease, and twice as likely to suffer from depression and digestive disorders like celiac disease and irritable bowel syndrome (IBS).

They are also more prone to certain types of athletic injuries with tendinitis, patella-femoral syndrome, ACL tears, stress fractures, and plantar fasciitis leading the list. They're injured more often, too. According to research done at the University of Alberta, female athletes experience dramatically higher rates of musculoskeletal injuries because the training programs designed for them are built on data gathered from studying young, adult males. They don't take the anatomical, physiological, or biological differences between men and women into account.

While women now represent more than half of all competitive sports participants, scientific studies that investigate athletic injury and performance issues utilize male subjects a full 97 to 98% of the time; that means only two to three percent of the subjects are female. Despite their high level of participation in sports, there's a lack of female-specific data in the realm of exercise science research.

The hormonal variances that are inextricably linked to the menstrual cycle complicate the scientific study participant selection process, which is the primary reason why many researchers find it difficult to include women in their work. Every potential female research subject is required to undergo both hormone and pregnancy testing. And studies can only be done on women who are not taking birth control pills. These factors not only decrease the total pool of qualified study participants, they increase research-related time and costs.

For at least the foreseeable future, female athletes won't have a lot of gender-specific data to make educated and informed choices on how to train or what to eat for peak health and performance. The needs of the female athlete struggling with poor performance, chronic illness, or recurring injuries are even less understood. And insights into how and why some women ultimately recover from these issues faster (and more permanently) than others remain (mostly) a mystery.

Age plays an obvious role in determining a woman's capacity for health, performance, and recovery. So do dietary and lifestyle choices. And while we can't stop the hands of time from turning, we do have a great deal of control over what we choose to eat or not to eat; how we exercise, manage our stress levels, and prioritize the importance of making health-enhancing lifestyle choices.

AN INTRODUCTION

This book was written to inform and inspire female athletes of all shapes and sizes, ages and ability levels. It was designed to provide an overview of the most common obstacles that prevent women from achieving optimal health and performance, and to offer some actionable insights into overcoming them.

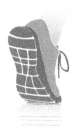

Obstacle One

An Energy Imbalance

Food Fundamentals

On the surface, we all know what food is—it's what we eat when we're hungry. But looking closer, we see that it's so much more. Food is the source of all the raw materials we need to build and repair our tissues, organs, and systems. Food is information, in the form of nutrients, that tells our cells what they should or shouldn't be doing. And food is fuel; it's the potential pool of energy we give our bodies to work with.

Food affects our physical and mental health, arguably more than any other lifestyle choice we make. Of course, dietary habits and food preferences can vary significantly from one woman to another. And given that our genealogy, biology, physiology, and psychology are all very different, that makes perfect sense. Despite the rise (and inevitable fall) of any given dietary trend, it's important to realize that there's no such thing as a one-size-fits-all formula for eating, moving, or living well.

The relationship between mind, body, and food is incredibly complex. While analyzing it lies beyond the scope of this book, we can explore the body's basic energy requirements and understand why satisfying them is so important for optimal health, performance, and recovery.

Compared to our hunting and gathering ancestors, most women in modern societies enjoy relatively easy access to an abundant supply of food. As a result, some end up struggling with health and performance issues that stem from eating too much and moving too little. But many fit, active women have an entirely different obstacle—a negative energy imbalance caused by eating too little and moving too much.

While being over or under weight is the most obvious indication of an energy imbalance, addressing and overcoming this obstacle is complex and involves more than just gaining or losing a few pounds.

Finding Your Balance

Energy balance plays a key role in determining something that's much more important than how much you weigh; it determines the strength or weakness of your underlying cellular health. When your energy balance is disrupted, everything from your strength, endurance, and immunity to your metabolism, mindset, and mood can be impaired.

When faced with an ongoing energy deficit, for example, the thyroid and adrenal glands will release hormones that slow metabolism down. This is because the female body has been programmed to reduce its expenditure of energy when a (real or perceived) scarcity threatens its survival. In fact, a chronic energy deficit is one of the primary reasons why women who follow calorie restriction diets often end up gaining—instead of losing—weight.

Are You Eating Enough?

It's not enough to rely on what the scale says or how your clothes fit. What matters most is how you feel. Do you have even, consistent energy throughout the day? Or do you experience troublesome high's and low's? Chronic under-eating leaves you more susceptible to suffering from hypoglycemia (low blood sugar), which can cause symptoms that range from hunger, unexplained sweating, and muscular weakness to dizziness, anxiety, and confusion.

Have you ever heard the term *hangry* **before?** It's urban slang used to describe the feelings of anger and irritability that come from being really, really hungry. Even though the term is made up, there's plenty of hard-core, scientific evidence supporting the validity of this volatile emotional state caused by an insufficient food intake. The brain depends on a steady supply of glucose to function optimally. When blood sugar levels fall too low, one of the first cognitive processes to suffer is self-control. A lack of self-control can make paying attention, regulating emotions, coping with stress, and refraining from impulsive actions very difficult.

 The body can also express its need for more energy in a number of other, often-unexpected ways.

Are you often constipated? Chronic under-eating may be the culprit since an ongoing energy deficit can negatively impact thyroid hormone production. Constipation is a common symptom of hypothyroidism (low thyroid function) since thyroid hormone controls peristalsis—the wave-like contractions in the intestines that keep the digestive process working smoothly and efficiently. When thyroid hormone levels drop, the entire elimination process slows causing chronic constipation.

Do you sleep well? Insomnia and other sleep-related disturbances are a common complaint among female athletes. But poor sleep is particularly problematic for those who run on empty. As blood sugar levels naturally decline during the night, the liver must release stored glucose in order to support the body's basic physiological functions. If your energy balance is consistently negative, your liver won't have enough fuel to work with. In a low blood sugar emergency, adrenaline and cortisol rush to the scene, turning on gluconeogenesis—the production of new glucose from stored energy. This sudden spike in stress hormone levels can wake you, even from a sound sleep.

Do you frequently feel cold? An energy deficit can lower your body temperature. Without an adequate supply of energy, the body can't support thermogenesis—the natural production of body heat. A low insulin level can also lead to reduced thermogenesis and a low body temperature so women who follow a very low-carbohydrate diet may often feel cold, too.

Have you experienced unexplained hair loss? Hair loss is one of the first signs of a nutritional deficiency and/or hormonal imbalance created by an energy insufficiency. It's also a very common symptom of hypothyroidism, which can be the end result of a long-term energy imbalance.

Do you have lots of headaches? Not all women experience hunger in the same way. Instead of a growling stomach, hunger can sometimes surface as a headache. Hunger-related headaches are a clear sign that the body doesn't have enough available energy to meet its immediate needs. The drop in blood sugar and subsequent release of stress hormones (adrenaline and cortisol) that trigger a hunger headache can also cause anxiety, irritability, confusion, and fatigue. Adrenaline and cortisol will also increase when a woman is dehydrated or suffering from a lack of sleep.

Why don't all women feel hungry when they need to eat?

There are a number of reasons, but stress is the most common one. While some women feel like nibbling on something to ease their anxiety, others respond to stress by unconsciously putting their appetites on hold. Both physical and mental stress can stimulate the release of corticotropin (an appetite-suppressing hormone) and epinephrine (a fight or flight hormone that decreases hunger).

Iron deficiency can also blunt the appetite. The body needs iron in order to make hemoglobin, a complex protein found in the red blood cells that's responsible for oxygen transport. Low iron contributes to low hemoglobin which, in turn, reduces the amount of ghrelin (the hunger hormone responsible for regulating the appetite) and insulin (which stimulates the body's need to eat) released in the body.

A lack of vitamin B12 rich foods (like red meat) can also suppress hunger. And certain medications (both prescribed and over-the-counter) can weaken the appetite as well. The most common offenders are acetaminophen, codeine, muscle relaxants, antifungals, antidepressants, antibiotics, and diuretics.

How Much Should You be Eating?

Determining the number of calories your body needs on a daily basis for optimal health, performance, and recovery can be a little tricky. Among the many variables to consider, it's important to evaluate how much of what kind of food you eat as well as the type, frequency, and intensity of any physical activity you do.

While it's difficult to determine your exact calorie requirements, there are some ways to get a fairly accurate estimate of your daily minimum. If you enjoy math, you could use the Harris-Benedict Equation. It offers a reasonable estimate of your basal metabolic rate or BMR—the minimum number of calories your body needs to perform its basic, life-sustaining functions.

$$BMR = 655.1 + (4.35 \times \text{weight in pounds}) + (4.7 \times \text{height in inches}) - (4.7 \times \text{age})$$

Doing the math results in a caloric estimate that has about a 10% margin of error, which might not seem like much. But if your estimated BMR is 1,700 calories a day, your actual need will lie somewhere between 1,530 and 1,870.

Multiplied on a daily, weekly, and monthly basis, it's easy to see why relying on this formula can lead to an energy imbalance. And remember, this equation doesn't take your activity level or health status into account.

Another way to get an idea of the minimum number of calories you should be eating is to simply multiply your ideal body weight by 10. Again, it's important to note that this quick estimate applies only to a sedentary body; it doesn't take the additional energy demands of physical activity or injury recovery into account.

While these formulas can help you begin to assess your energy needs, monitoring your body for clues that come in the form of hunger, fatigue, headaches, anxiety, weight gain, weight loss, digestive difficulties, fitness declines, or delayed recovery will ultimately be more useful.

If you're trying to gain or lose weight, an energy balance equation can offer some guidance. But it won't provide you with any insights into your body composition (the relative percentages of fat, muscle, bone, and water you're made of) or the status of your underlying cellular health (which determines your overall capacity for health, performance, and recovery).

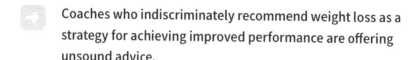

Coaches who indiscriminately recommend weight loss as a strategy for achieving improved performance are offering unsound advice.

Theoretically, weighing less can lead to an improved VO2 max (the amount of oxygen a woman's body utilizes during movement). Regardless of how much a woman weighs, her heart and lungs remain consistently proficient at delivering oxygen-rich blood to her muscles. When her muscles are required to move less mass, her efficiency (and speed) will naturally increase. However, the long-term health risks outweigh the short-term benefits of any training program that includes arbitrary weight loss goals.

Since no two women have the same biological, physiological or psychological history, it's virtually impossible to determine the ideal weight any female athlete should strive to achieve. Even with extensive laboratory testing, the number of possible interactions among the dozens of variables involved mean that weight loss won't guarantee optimal athletic performance.

In fact, when the female body is deprived of essential nutrients its capacity for consistent energy production, hormonal function, and neurological adaptation can be compromised. The resulting insufficiencies and imbalances do not contribute to any long-term health or performance gains. Rather, they become stumbling blocks that contribute to a significantly increased risk of bone, muscle, and connective tissue injuries—and to debilitating psychological distress.

Calorie restriction can also be counterproductive because it activates a woman's fight or flight response. A chronic food scarcity triggers the body's innate, protective drive to store the calories it receives as fat—the safe and reliable form of fuel it depends on for emergency survival.

The Calorie Conundrum

Determining the caloric content of any given food isn't as simple as you might think. In fact, it can't even be done without the use of a calorimeter—a piece of laboratory equipment that heats a food until it burns and releases all its energy. This energy is measured in calories. One calorie is the amount of energy it takes to heat one kilogram of water one degree Celsius.

Of course, the female body is a lot more complicated than an expensive oven. When food is burned in a lab, it surrenders its calories within a few seconds. The actual journey food takes from the dinner plate to the toilet bowl lasts about a day on average, but it can range from eight to 80 hours depending on the woman.

Our attachment to counting calories incorrectly assumes that they are all created equal. It's often said that we shouldn't "compare apples to oranges" because they aren't the same. Neither are the calories found in cookies and chicken. A calorie of carbohydrate and a calorie of protein both contain the same amount of stored energy so they perform identically when burned in a lab. But when those two different types of calories are put into real bodies, they behave quite differently.

In 1918, the first book on nutrition was published in America. It was based on the notion that following a healthy diet could be achieved by simply adding and subtracting calories. In her book, *Diet and Health*, Lulu Peters wrote, "You may eat just what you like—candy, pie, cake, fat, meat, butter, cream—but count your calories!" The book quickly became a national best-seller.

By the 1930s, calorie counting became entrenched in both the American public's mind and the U.S. government's policy. Its exclusive focus on the *energy* content of food (quantity), rather than its *nutrient* content (quality) went virtually unchallenged.

By the 1960s, rising incomes and more women in the workforce meant that people were dining out more often and buying more packaged foods, so they naturally wanted more information about what they were eating. Nutritional values were placed on food labels, but they weren't very consistent. It wasn't until 1990 that food labelling became standardized and mandatory in America.

Unfortunately, our food labels still aren't entirely accurate.

According to Susan Roberts, a nutritionist at Tufts University in Boston, the labels on most American packaged foods miss their true calorie counts by an average of 8%. Government regulations allow for the understatement of calories by up to 20%. So while the columns of numbers found on food labels might seem scientific, they're really only approximations.

 While the long-accepted formula of calories in/calories out isn't exactly wrong, it is more complicated.

The way any given food is prepared, for example, can affect the body's ability to utilize it. Chopping and grinding food takes care of some digestive work, making more calories available to your body by ripping apart cell walls even before it's chewed.

Similarly, how quickly or slowly you eat can make a difference in how well you digest and utilize your food. While some vitamins are better absorbed from raw food, most macronutrients (proteins, fats, and carbohydrates) are absorbed faster, and more completely, when they're cooked. In fact, research indicates that cooking increases the proportion of food digested in the stomach and small intestine from 50 to 95%.

Genetic differences are another variable that can affect digestion and assimilation. Some women are born with intestines that are up to 50% longer than others, which gives their digestive system additional time to extract more calories from the food they eat. Women with shorter intestines will absorb fewer calories and have a harder time gaining and maintaining weight.

Because muscle burns more energy than fat, differences in body composition translate into differences in how many calories a woman's body will burn. And because it takes energy to process and store energy, the thermic effect of different foods (with their different macronutrient profiles) can affect the body's digestion and metabolism.

In addition, a growing body of research suggests that no two women will metabolize their food in the same way with all other factors being equal. These digestive differences are attributed to the unique blend and balance of intestinal flora each woman houses in her gut. If you and I were to consume identical meals, the nutrients they contain would be processed and utilized differently.

Should You Blame Your Metabolism?

When faced with an energy imbalance, the default is often to blame either a sluggish or an overactive metabolism.

Metabolism is a term that's commonly used to describe how quickly or easily the body burns calories, but it's better thought of as the 'engine' that powers everything we think and do. While one woman's metabolism might run a little 'hotter' or 'cooler' than another's, research studies suggest that there's a negligible difference in the relative number of calories each one burns.

It is true that men have a faster metabolism than women (because they typically carry less fat and have more lean muscle); but it slows down for both genders after the age of 40. The female metabolism also slows with decreased estrogen levels during menopause, and as a result of age-related muscle loss.

Other Factors Affecting Metabolism

We all know that exercise requires energy, and that we need more energy when we're actively training than when we're not. While movement-related activity consumes 10 to 15% of a minimally active woman's day-to-day energy budget, it can account for 30% or more of that used by an athlete. Higher-intensity workouts create a higher demand for energy, both during and after activity. And exercise that involves a greater range and intensity of muscular challenge—like full-body strength training—not only requires more energy, but builds metabolic might. That means 30 minutes of hard work in the weight room can do more to improve your metabolic health than an hour of easy running.

Metabolism can also be affected by an injury. While the initial phase of recovery is often a primary focus, the subsequent stages of healing are actually more energy-intensive. During proliferation (when damaged tissue is temporarily replaced) and remodeling (when tissue replacement becomes permanent), a woman's basal metabolic rate may increase by 15 to 50% depending on the severity of her trauma. A common sports injury might raise her BMR by 15 to 20%; a major surgery by 50%. Comparatively speaking, an athlete will need fewer calories while she's recovering from an injury or surgery than when training and competing, but more than what's necessary for supporting her basic metabolic requirements.

Research indicates that a continuous energy deficit can reduce the body's BMR by 5 to 15%. An insufficient calorie intake acts as a red flag warning for the 'primitive brain' to protect the body from deprivation and scarcity. It accomplishes this task by slowing down metabolism—the body's energy output.

When the thyroid gland inevitably receives an alert, it downregulates its systems in an effort to limit fertility (since having a baby to feed during a famine is not a fantastic idea). Over time, a negative energy imbalance will also make the female body increasingly prone to fatigue, injury, cognitive difficulties, and a weakened immune response. An energy deficit will also impair a woman's ability to recover quickly and/or completely from any illness or injury.

Metabolic Factors Affecting Weight Loss

Stubborn weight loss (in the absence of an identified energy imbalance) is a pervasive problem, even for fit female athletes (especially those over the age of 40). The four most common reasons why many active women struggle to achieve and maintain a lean body composition include:

1. Nutrient Deficiencies. Studies show that macronutrient (fat, protein, and carbohydrate) and/or micronutrient (vitamin and mineral) imbalances are a large and growing problem for men and women alike. In fact, more than 30% of the U.S. population doesn't consume enough magnesium or vitamins C, E, and A to support optimal metabolic health. More than 80% have low vitamin D3 levels, and nine out of 10 are deficient in omega-3 fatty acids which, among other things, help reduce inflammation and stabilize blood sugar. D3 and omega-3s also drive the body's metabolic preference for either accessing and utilizing or producing and storing fat.

2. Microbiome Imbalances. We have more than a thousand different species of bacteria living inside our intestinal tracts. From both animal and human studies, we know that these bacteria play a significant role in determining the status of our metabolic health. Some bacteria extract more energy from food, leading to weight gain; others extract less, leading to weight loss. In fact, studies have shown that implanting the gut bacteria from a thin mouse into a fat mouse consistently leads to dramatic weight loss.

In addition, some bacteria cause systemic inflammation which contributes to both insulin resistance (faulty blood sugar processing) and fat production, regardless of caloric intake. If you are struggling with stubborn weight loss, assessing and addressing the health of your intestinal microbiome should be a top priority.

3. Systemic Inflammation. Scientists have identified systemic inflammation (lasting inflammation that affects the entire body) as the root cause of most modern, chronic disease. In fact, allergies, asthma, arthritis, autism, autoimmune dysfunction, cancer, dementia, depression, diabetes, heart disease, and obesity all begin with systemic inflammation.

Because fat cells (particularly those found in the body's midsection) produce inflammatory molecules that promote fat production and storage, a little excess body fat can turn into a lot of excess body fat—even in the absence of an energy imbalance. Identifying the hidden source (or sources) of systemic inflammation is often critical for women who struggle to get and stay lean.

4. Environmental Toxins. Many conventional doctors overlook the damaging impact toxins have on our overall health and wellbeing. While detoxification is a naturally and regularly occurring physiological process, the body's innate ability to detoxify can be hindered by many factors including the long-term use of medications and the ever-increasing number of chemicals found in our food, air, water, and homes.

These harmful substances include plastics, pesticides, and preservatives. And heavy metals like lead, mercury, arsenic, and aluminium. We are exposed to them when we use conventional cosmetics and cleaning solutions or unknowingly come in contact with any of the 80,000 chemical compounds that have been created since the industrial revolution. Certain toxins have been shown to interfere with metabolism and cause weight gain, even in the absence of excess calories. They are appropriately referred to as *obesogens*.

Reducing your body's total toxic load is both important and possible, which is why Chapter Seven has been dedicated entirely to this topic.

Evaluating Energy

If you've ever read a fitness nutrition book or blog, you've probably heard the term 'macros' thrown around. It's short for macronutrients and it refers to carbohydrates, fats, and proteins—the three essential energy components of the human diet.

Since the energy macronutrients contain provide the foundation on which a lean, strong, and resilient body is built, it's important to understand their structure and function. So let's take an in-depth look at each of the three macronutrients. And let's begin with the controversial carbohydrate.

Carbohydrates

While different types of carbohydrates from breads and blueberries to beets and black beans are all digested and utilized a little differently, they're all made of carbon and hydrogen molecules which are eventually broken down into glucose—the simplest form of sugar the body can use. As soon as the body finishes converting dietary carbohydrates into glucose, this simple fuel is either burned for immediate energy, stored in the liver or muscles as glycogen (the storage form of glucose), or converted into triglycerides (the storage form of fat).

Simple carbohydrates are swiftly absorbed into the bloodstream, providing a quick boost of energy. The body absorbs the sugar found in a can of soda at a rate of 30 calories per minute. Complex carbohydrates (like sweet potatoes) are absorbed at a rate of two calories per minute. The difference in the absorption rates matters because the presence of a large amount of sugar in the bloodstream triggers the rapid release of insulin—a hormone that carries the sugar out of the bloodstream and into the cells.

Once the cells have taken in all the glycogen they can handle, the liver accepts as much as it can. Any additional amount is stored as fat.

Unfortunately, this isn't your ordinary, run-of-the-mill form of body fat (the often-unwanted but inactive variety that takes up residence in the thighs, hips, and waist). It's inflammatory fat—the invisible fat that infiltrates the intestinal lining, the liver, the kidneys, and even the heart. Inflammatory fat is metabolically active; it creates and releases cellular signaling molecules called cytokines.

Cytokines fuel the spread of chronic inflammation, robbing the body of its full health, performance, and recovery potential.

Why is the body in such a rush to get rid of glucose?

Because high blood sugar can be a big problem. A healthy woman should have only a teaspoon of glucose circulating in her bloodstream at any given time. Any additional amount would result in *hyperglycemia* (excess blood sugar) which, over time, would lead to diabetes and impair the functional health of every organ and system in her body. *Hypoglycemia* is caused by an insufficient (less than a teaspoon) amount of glucose circulating in the bloodstream. Chronic bouts of low blood sugar can wreak havoc on a woman's hormonal, digestive, and central nervous systems, compromising every aspect of her health, performance, and recovery.

The type, length, and intensity of a woman's training program will play a key role in determining how quickly her body burns through its blood glucose supply. From a health perspective, even the fastest and fittest of athletes can benefit from reducing their dependence on carbohydrates as a primary source of fuel.

Achieving and maintaining a healthy blood sugar level is a delicate balancing act. But from an evolutionary perspective, it's one that has been managed extremely well for thousands of years by the body's internal, metabolic processes, not from the constant intake of a large amount of dietary carbohydrates.

From an ancestral standpoint, excessive carbohydrate consumption wasn't a problem until quite recently. Grains, for example, were introduced into the human diet a mere 10,000 years ago—a few seconds when considered in an evolutionary context. In the United States, the Standard American Diet (SAD) is now dominated by simple carbohydrates in the form of processed grains and sugars. The massive increase in their consumption over the past 100 years has been definitively linked to the onset of most 'modern' chronic disease.

Because the high glucose levels caused by excessive carbohydrate consumption contribute to the production of inflammatory fat, they also contribute to systemic inflammation. To some extent, inflammation is a healthy, physiological response; it offers evidence that our immune system is working.

Most female athletes are always experiencing some degree of chronic, low-grade inflammation in their bodies. When fed by excessive glucose, however, it can flare and spread.

Systemic inflammation is increasingly being identified as a contributing factor in the onset of a number of orthopedic conditions including osteoarthritis, which makes sense given that repetitive rise and fall of blood sugar can literally wear a woman's body down. Insulin instability accelerates the rate of cellular division, which ultimately leads to premature aging and a significantly increased risk of both illness and injury.

It can also lead to insulin resistance, a condition in which the body can no longer process blood sugar properly. Cells become insulin-resistant when the amount of glucose they are required to process leads to exhaustion. Tired and overworked, they becomes less and less efficient at performing their sugar-processing function. In an effort to correct the resulting blood sugar surplus, the body defaults to producing more fat which gives glucose—in the form of triglycerides—a place to go.

Clearly, high blood sugar isn't a good thing. What happens if it drops too low?

While the initial symptom of low blood sugar is typically hunger, some women experience headaches, fatigue, sugar cravings, dizziness, or a decrease in focus and concentration first. If and when these symptoms are ignored and a woman's energy need remains unmet, she will likely end up experiencing what many athletes refer to as "hitting the wall" or "bonking."

The fear of bonking has caused many female athletes to become overly dependent on carbohydrate-based fuel. It's important to note, however, that low blood sugar is a relatively easy problem for the body to solve. Even in the complete absence of dietary carbohydrates, the metabolic processes of *gluconeogenesis* (the creation of glucose from a non-carbohydrate source) and *ketosis* (the burning of fat as a primary source of energy) can adequately meet the body's energy needs.

In all fairness, it's important to acknowledge that the brain does rely on glucose to function (although it doesn't absolutely have to). And it's the preferred form of fuel for muscles exercising at medium to high intensity. For these reasons, conventional dietary recommendations for athletes are typically skewed toward a higher carbohydrate intake.

 The body's ability to store glucose, however, is extremely limited. Since it can only be stored in small amounts and must be used quickly, it needs to be replenished frequently. This makes carbohydrates a very inefficient form of fuel.

How many carbohydrates does the average female athlete need?

The answer can vary greatly from one woman to another. Her age and activity level are key considerations. So are her individual circumstances. For example, an athlete who is suffering from a functional adrenal weakness or recovering from an injury or illness will most certainly need a larger supply of easily and quickly digested carbohydrate energy.

As a very general guideline, the brain and other key organs require about 150 grams of carbohydrate a day to sustain their basic functions. Becoming a fat-adapted athlete, however, can significantly reduce the body's reliance on glucose as a primary source of fuel. In fact, an extremely limited carbohydrate intake (50 or fewer grams a day) will force the body into the metabolic state known as ketosis, when fat is burned as a primary source of fuel.

The Case Against Carbohydrate Loading

Carbohydrates supply the body's metabolic fire with kindling. They ignite and burn quickly, but need to be continuously replaced and end up creating a lot of unwanted metabolic waste (like ash from burning paper). Relying on a constant supply of carbohydrates as a primary source of energy is not only inefficient, but unhealthy.

The body is, however, incredibly resilient; it can adapt to running pretty well on carbohydrate-based fuel. This is one of the reasons why endurance athletes who rely on carbohydrates for energy feel the need to 'carb load.' Over time, they have conditioned their bodies to store more carbohydrates as glycogen in order to satisfy an increased energy need. Even with this expanded storage capacity, however, the practice of carbohydrate loading is still ineffective.

The concept of carbohydrate loading is flawed from both a quantitative and a qualitative perspective. Fueling the body with a large-amount of carbohydrates is a lot like filling your car with a cheaper gas that gets fewer miles per gallon. During an endurance event, the athletes who are dependent on this type of inferior fuel won't arrive at their intended destination (the finish) without carrying some additional 'tanks' of fuel (extra carbohydrates). The better solution is to use a higher-quality fuel to begin with.

The fat-adapted athlete has essentially trained her body to utilize its own fat stores for energy. As a result, her physical and mental output will remain stable, even if she begins to feel a little hungry. Like the working embers left from a hot fire, her body's internal engine will continue to run smoothly and efficiently by utilizing fat to create steady, slow-burning energy. It will no longer have to be completely dependent on quick-burning carbohydrates for fuel.

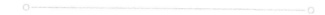

The Glycemic Index

The more rapidly a carbohydrate is broken down, the higher it's *glycemic index* or GI—the relative ranking of a carbohydrate based on how quickly it increases blood glucose (and insulin). Carbohydrates with a low GI value are metabolized slowly, which means they increase blood sugar and insulin gradually. In general, carbohydrates that are less processed and higher in fiber will contain a more complex carbohydrate structure and lower GI. A whole orange, for example, takes time to eat and is rich in fiber so it has a much lower glycemic index than a glass of orange juice, which contains the same amount of carbohydrates found in two or three oranges and can be consumed in less than a minute. Steel cut oats (which require 30 minutes of stove top cooking and are rich in fiber) have a very low GI; rolled oats (which have less fiber and fewer nutrients) have a moderate index, and instant oats (which have the least amount of fiber and nutrients) are scored very high.

Because complex carbohydrates are digested more slowly, their energy is released more evenly which keeps us fueled (and full) longer. Fresh, whole vegetables, some fruits, and certain unrefined, 'ancient' grains are the preferred sources. While an extensive list of low-glycemic foods can be found online, here's an abbreviated list of the top choices in each category:

Low-Glycemic Vegetables

Asparagus	Celery	Peppers
Broccoli	Green Beans	Salad Greens
Brussels Sprouts	Leafy Greens	Sugar Snap Peas
Cabbage	Onions	Sweet Potatoes
Cauliflower	Pea Pods	Squashes

Low-Glycemic Fruits

Apricots	Nectarines	Pears
Blueberries	Oranges	Strawberries
Cantaloupe	Peaches	Watermelon
Grapefruit		

Low-Glycemic Grains

Barley	Steel Cut Oats	Rye
Black Rice	Quinoa	Wild Rice
Buckwheat		

Are gluten-free foods less glycemic?

No. In fact, many gluten-free foods have a very high glycemic index. While following a gluten-free diet can offer many health and performance-related benefits, be wary of products that feature simple, processed grains, starches, and sugars—especially as a first ingredient. Some gluten-free breads, cereals, and pastas can actually raise blood glucose and insulin levels higher than a *Milky Way* or *Snickers Bar*. The candy bars contain enough protein and fat to slow the digestion and absorption of their sugar content down.

Speaking of Sugar

Sugar is the generic name for sweet-tasting, soluble carbohydrates. Simple sugars (monosaccharides) include glucose, fructose, and galactose. Compound sugars (called disaccharides or double sugars) are molecules composed of two monosaccharides. Common examples of compound sugars include table sugar (or sucrose), lactose, and maltose.

Longer chains of sugar molecules (known as oligosaccharides or polysaccharides) may have a sweet taste but aren't really sugars. Examples of these include inulin, glycerol, and sugar alcohols such as erythritol, xylitol, and maltitol. Since sugar alcohols are not absorbed completely in the small intestine, they contain fewer calories and have a significantly lower impact on blood glucose levels. This makes them a popular choice for diabetics and/or those adhering to a low-carbohydrate diet.

True sugars are found in the tissues of most plants. Most fruits offer an abundant supply of simple sugars. Sucrose is especially concentrated in sugarcane and sugar beet, making them ideal for processing into commercially refined sugar. Maltose can be produced by malting (germinating) grain. Lactose is the only sugar that cannot be extracted from plants. It can only be found in milk (including human breast milk) and in some dairy products. The cheapest source of sugar is corn syrup, which is industrially produced by converting corn starch into sugars such as maltose, fructose, and glucose.

The average American consumes about 53 pounds of sugar each year, which adds up to about 260 calories per day. As sugar consumption increased in the latter part of the 20th century, researchers began to look at the effects of a high-sugar diet. They wanted to know if sugar, especially refined sugar, was damaging to human health. The results of their long-term studies are fairly conclusive. The excessive consumption of sugar has been implicated in the onset of obesity, diabetes, cardiovascular disease, immune dysfunction, dementia, premature aging, and (of course) tooth decay.

It's important to note, however, that different types of sugar can have different effects on the body. And that their relative health consequences can vary greatly depending on how complex, sweet, processed, or nutrient-dense a sugar is.

While less-processed sugars such as yacon syrup, coconut palm sugar, raw honey, maple and barley malt syrups, and unrefined cane sugar are all less glycemic than refined white sugar, they should still be consumed in moderation. Agave syrup has been successfully marketed as a healthier sweetener, but it creates some of the worst insulin-spiking side effects of any 'natural' sweetener currently being sold.

Beware of Fructose. Because fructose has a lesser impact on blood sugar levels, many health professionals recommend it as a 'safe' sweetener, particularly for those with type 2 diabetes. Glucose and fructose, however, are metabolized very differently by the body. While every cell in the body can use glucose, the liver is the only organ that can process fructose in any significant amount. Regularly eating foods that are high in fructose will overload the liver, prompting the body to convert any excess into fat.

A century ago, the average American consumed about 15 grams of fructose a day, which came from eating fresh fruits and vegetables that also contain fiber, vitamins, minerals, enzymes, and other beneficial nutrients. This amount has now increased to roughly 75 grams of fructose a day, with much of it being consumed in the form of high-fructose corn syrup (HFCS). Studies have confirmed that HFCS is turned into inflammatory fat far more rapidly than any other type of sugar. In fact, the massive increase in U.S. obesity and diabetes rates directly parallels the introduction of high-fructose corn syrup in soft drinks during the late 1970s.

Large amounts of fructose can be found in more than just high-fructose corn syrup. Agave nectar, for example, is 90% fructose. Regular corn syrup, honey, cane sugar, maple syrup, and many fruits are just 50% fructose by comparison.

What about calorie-free sweeteners? Zero-calorie sweeteners do not have a glycemic index; they don't raise blood sugar at all. It doesn't mater if the sweetener is natural (like stevia or monk fruit) or artificial (like saccharin or aspartame) Still, the human body is hard-wired to react to the taste of sweet things.

Studies have shown that insulin is secreted by the pancreas soon after a sweet taste is experienced on the tongue, whether the substance contains calories or not. The body is essentially fooled by no-calorie sweeteners. When the glucose it has been programmed to expect isn't delivered, a sharp increase in appetite is often experienced as a rebound effect. Numerous studies prove that the use of calorie-free sweeteners does not aid weight loss. This may explain why.

 At this point, it should be clear to see that not all carbohydrates are created equal. And that different types of carbohydrates can have different effects on our overall health and wellbeing.

Starches, for example, are a type of carbohydrate composed of long chains of glucose molecules that are easily broken down and readily absorbed by the small intestine. Resistant starches are different. They take they express route through the small intestine, completely undigested, before being transferred to the large intestine for elimination. They are called *resistant starches* due to their unique ability to resist digestion.

Once they enter the large intestine, however, resistant starches can be broken down and used as fuel by the beneficial bacteria living there. This makes them an excellent *prebiotic* food source. Resistant starches are also *symbiotic*; they help intestinal bacteria interact better together. And they can be turned into short-chain fatty acids like butyrate which can heal the gut lining and support improved intestinal health.

Mounting research suggests that the activity of resistant starches can effectively enhance the actions of our intestinal bacteria, improving insulin sensitivity (the cells' readiness to accept and process blood sugar) and decreasing systemic inflammation. The short-chain fatty acids they provide for can support detoxification, increase nutrient and mineral absorption, and boost both the production and efficacy of immune cells.

Some of the best sources of resistant starch include:

- Cashew nuts
- Cooked adzuki, black, red, white beans, and lentils
- Cooked and cooled heirloom potatoes
- Cooked and cooled white rice
- Sweet potatoes and yams
- Polenta
- Cassava starch
- Plantain flour
- Raw mung beans
- Rye bread

Fats

While carbohydrates provide fast-burning energy, fats are an exceptionally fuel-efficient macronutrient that consistently deliver the slow-burning energy we need to fuel our everyday activities and/or longer, slower endurance activity.

Remember the low-fat craze of the 1980s and 90s? Fat—especially saturated fat—was demonized and unfairly blamed for the skyrocketing incidence of chronic illness. We now know that large amounts of sugar and/or processed carbohydrates are the real health hazard.

Eating more of the right kind of fat can:

- Increase the burning of excess body fat
- Improve digestion and elimination

- Reduce sugar and carbohydrate cravings
- Enhance both physical and mental performance
- Promote healing and recovery

From a purely evolutionary perspective, fat has been the primary fuel source responsible for sustaining human life. Since this energy-dense macronutrient supported the growth and development of a more complex brain, fat is literally what made us human. Mastering the use of fire for cooking animal meat greatly reduced the incidence of foodborne illnesses, allowing for its safe and consistent consumption. The high-fat elements of regular meat intake provided an exceptional source of nourishment to the brain, allowing our intellectual capabilities to rise above those of our predominantly vegetarian great ape cousins.

The building of a campfire provides a useful analogy for examining how our bodies burn fats and carbohydrates differently. In order to create an efficient and long-lasting fire, we need substantial, slow-burning logs. While we might use kindling to get our fire started, it would be inefficient to build it entirely out of twigs and newspaper. We would have to feed the fire constantly in order to keep it going. It would never get very hot and all of the ash (metabolic waste) it produced would be unpleasant and annoying. Carbohydrates are like twigs and newspaper; fats are like slow-burning logs.

In addition to being a longer, slower, and cleaner source of energy, fats are necessary for healthy (meaning flexible) cellular membranes. They provide the raw materials for many hormones while helping to regulate the function of several others. They assist in the transport and delivery of fat-soluble vitamins (like A, D3, K2, and E). Although we can make most of our own fatty acids, dietary fats provide us with the two critically essential ones we can't make—linolenic acid (an omega-3 fat) and linoleic acid (an omega-6 fat).

Fats are organic molecules made up of carbon and hydrogen elements joined together in larger groups called hydrocarbons. The arrangement of these hydrocarbon chains determines the fat type. The simplest unit of fat is the fatty acid.

Fatty acids are made up of simple hydrocarbon chains with open spaces that provide hydrogen atoms with a place to dock and bond. The more hydrogen atoms bonded to a chain, the more saturated the fat. Like dietary carbohydrates, dietary fats also come in different forms, each with their own health-enhancing (or reducing) effects.

Saturated fats (like coconut oil, butter, or palm oil) are easily identified because they are solid or semi-solid at room temperature. Since there are no empty spaces on their chains for any additional hydrogen atoms to bond, saturated fats are chemically stable. They don't oxidize or become damaged by interacting with oxygen easily. It makes sense that foods high in saturated fats thrive in warm climates; they have evolved and adapted to being more impervious to the damaging effects of heat.

Keep in mind that this type of naturally occurring saturation is very unlike that found in artificially saturated trans fats. These faux fats are created when hydrogen atoms are forced onto the available bonding sites of an unsaturated (liquid at room temperature) fat until it becomes solid. This industrial process is known as hydrogenation. Hydrogenation maximizes a product's profitability by prolonging its shelf life (at the expense of our health). Since trans fats have an abnormally rigid structure, the body can't process them like a natural fat. Research has shown that just one meal with a high trans fat content can negatively affect vascular function and blood vessel elasticity.

If some hydrogen bonding sites remain open, the resulting fat is considered unsaturated. The least-saturated fats include the anti-inflammatory omega-3 and the pro-inflammatory omega-6. Anthropological research suggests that our hunter-gatherer ancestors (who did not suffer from any form of inflammatory disease) consumed omega-6 and omega-3 fats in a ratio of roughly 1:1. Today, the ratio found in a typical American diet is somewhere between 10:1 and 30:1. When you consider that corn oil (prevalent in processed foods) has a ratio of 46:1, it's not that difficult to understand why fatty acid imbalances and chronic, inflammatory diseases have become so common. Since many female athletes are constantly battling the effects of chronic inflammation, particular attention should be given to maintaining a well-balanced unsaturated fat intake.

 The take home point is that there are bad fats (those that cause degenerative disease) and good fats (those we need for optimum health and performance).

In general, good fats are high in omega-3 fatty acids. They include the monounsaturates found in nuts, avocados, coconut products, and olive oil; the polyunsaturates found primarily in fish; and the saturated from grass-fed meats, coconut, and dairy products.

In addition to helping reduce chronic inflammation, the omega-3's act as a natural blood thinner promoting optimal brain function and oxygen delivery. Omega-3's are also very flexible, which allows them to be easily incorporated into our cellular membranes. The downside of this flexibility is that they are very susceptible to being damaged by high temperatures and light. Unlike the heat-hardy saturated fats, the omega-3 fats which include cold-water fish (such as salmon and sardines) and seeds (like flax and chia) are the product of colder environments.

But even the healthiest of fats can't be eaten in unlimited amounts; they are energy-dense and we still need to strive for an optimal energy balance. But good fats should be eaten regularly for optimal health, performance, and recovery. This may require a 180-degree shift in thinking, but the next time you butter a bite of bread, remember that the butter is the most nourishing part.

Bad fats are those that contain a disproportionately large amount of omega-6 fatty acids; they are typically sourced from plants (especially corn, soy, and canola), and are easily damaged by heat. While we need some omega-6 fats, especially for the formation of a bioactive fat called gamma linolenic acid which promotes youthful skin, a normal menstrual cycle, and a healthy metabolism, an excessive omega-6 fat intake leads to the onset of chronic inflammation.

Given what you now know, you may be questioning the American Heart Association's recommendation that adults limit their daily intake of calories from saturated fats to no more than 6%. In the interest of lowering blood cholesterol levels, they encourage the use of unsaturated vegetable oils instead. But swapping bad fats for good fats will not only jeopardize a woman's overall health and performance, it will increase her risk of suffering from a chronic disease.

 Cholesterol isn't the 'bad guy.' In fact, it's essential for optimal female health, performance, and recovery.

While we've been told to avoid high-cholesterol foods for many years, those days may soon be coming to an end. The vast amount of research pinpointing cholesterol as the root cause of chronic disease is, in fact, based on bad science. Concluding that cholesterol causes heart disease is a lot like deciding that firefighters set fires. Cholesterol might be present at the scene, but that doesn't mean it's the source of the problem.

What exactly is cholesterol? It's a type of fat that's essential for many of the body's metabolic processes. It's the raw material from which estrogen, progesterone, testosterone, cortisol, and vitamin D3 are all made. It's also a key component of every cell membrane in the body, lending essential shape and support. And it's a necessity for neurological health. Although the brain accounts for just 2% of the body's weight, it contains 25% of its total cholesterol content. To function well, the brain depends on a steady supply of cholesterol.

Because cholesterol is a fat and fat doesn't dissolve in water, it can't travel through blood and into the brain on its own. It needs to be carried by a *lipoprotein* (a fat surrounded by a water-soluble protein shell), which can vary in density from being very low to very high. High-density lipoproteins (HDLs) are considered beneficial because they play a key role in transporting excess cholesterol from the cells to the liver for processing and elimination. Certain types of low-density lipoproteins (LDLs), however, can present a problem because they direct the deposit of cholesterol into the arteries where it can accumulate and compromise blood flow.

To function fully and efficiently, the body requires about 1,000 mg of cholesterol a day. And it carefully regulates the amount it needs. The body produces more cholesterol if and when dietary sources don't provide enough. It also creates HDLs to bind and eliminate any excess. When this process of 'checks and balances' begins to break down, simple carbohydrates are usually the cause. The most recent research confirms that a high-carbohydrate intake decreases HDLs (the good guys) and increases LDLs (the bad guys.)

When it comes to determining what amount of cholesterol in the bloodstream is considered healthy (or not), it's the density of the lipoproteins carrying the cholesterol that ultimately matters more than the total amount of cholesterol itself—unless that amount is very high (exceeding 300 ng/dl).

Unfortunately, most standard blood tests don't offer a comprehensive breakdown of lipoprotein densities. If you're working with standard laboratory results, it's important to note that a total cholesterol to HDL ratio (optimally less than 3:0) and triglyceride to HDL ratio (optimally less than 1:1) are both indicators of good lipoprotein and metabolic health.

While the cholesterol controversy in the realm of conventional medicine continues, here's something to consider: men and women with higher total cholesterol levels actually live longer. There are a number of possible explanations for this. We know that cholesterol is necessary for supporting healthy cellular and hormonal function. It plays a key role in promoting fat metabolism. And numerous studies show that it improves brain function while protecting the body from cancer, bacterial and viral infections, atherosclerosis, and aging.

Protein

Like carbohydrates and fats, proteins are made of carbon and hydrogen molecules that combine to form chains; they differ in that they also contain nitrogen. The amino acid is the smallest unit of the protein chain and the fundamental building block the body needs to create, maintain, and repair all of its tissues, organs, and systems. Amino acids also serve as a catalyst in every chemical process affecting our physical and mental function.

In total, the body requires 22 different amino acids. Eight are considered 'essential' because they need to come from a food or supplement. The essential amino acids (EAAs) include the branched-chain (leucine, isoleucine, and valine) along with lysine, phenylalanine, threonine, tryptophan, and methionine. In addition to the 12 non-essential amino acids the body can make, there are several conditionally essential amino acids that we can make (although less efficiently) when we're experiencing periods of increased physical stress. These include arginine, cysteine, glutamine, tyrosine, glycine, ornithine, proline, and serine.

 When it comes to selecting a source of dietary protein, always choose 'quality over quantity.'

Higher-quality proteins will naturally offer a larger and more well-balanced supply of the eight essential amino acids the body needs for energy, growth, and recovery. These *high-biological-value proteins* include grass-fed meats, wild-caught fish, free-range poultry, and organic, whole eggs. The body uses approximately 40% of these protein sources for anabolic (constructive) purposes, which include the conversion of food into living tissue.

Other dietary proteins have a less-than-optimal mix of essential amino acids. Whey, soy, casein, beans, nuts, and egg whites all have a much lower biological value. Only about 20% of their protein content can be used anabolically.

Even if it were possible to consume nothing but 'perfect' sources of protein, their efficient use could not be guaranteed. Stress, age, digestive inefficiencies, intestinal bacteria (biome) imbalances, the use of many medications, and high-heat cooking methods can limit the body's ability to fully digest, absorb, and utilize their essential amino acid components.

Another way we can judge the quality of a protein is by evaluating its NNU (net nitrogen utilization) which pinpoints how many of its nitrogen molecules are retained by the body (and used for anabolic purposes) as opposed to being catabolized (and used for energy). In a theoretically perfect protein, every single one of its essential amino acids would be used for construction and maintenance. This theoretically ideal protein would have an assigned NNU of 100%. Eggs occupy the first real position on the list with an NNU of 45%; grazed or pastured animal meat, 30%; protein powders, 18%.

Athletes know that their bodies need protein and most are conscientious about eating enough. Some even take the time to calculate their protein intake requirements based on their body weight and activity level. Unfortunately, the results of these calculations aren't very accurate because they don't account for the biological value of a particular protein source. Despite all the performance and recovery hype surrounding the use of supplemental protein bars and powders (with their low NNU value of 18%) their functional benefits literally don't add up.

Perhaps you're wondering how whole eggs could be such an excellent source of protein with their somewhat below average NNU of 45%. It's because proteins, in general, are 'costly' to consume; they require a lot more digestive energy than either fats or carbohydrates. So a considerable portion of the energy found in any kind of dietary protein is being skimmed off the top and used for its own processing.

How much protein should a woman eat?

It depends. In terms of quantity, the American College of Sports Medicine recommends .6 to .8 grams of protein per pound of lean body mass daily. The International Society of Sports Nutrition suggests a little more (.7 to .9 grams per pound). The application of these guidelines will vary based on a woman's activity level and general health status.

Because women weigh less than men, their total protein intake needs have historically been thought to be lower. More recent research, however, suggests that women actually need to eat a little more protein per pound of body weight since their naturally higher progesterone levels skew their protein metabolism more toward the catabolic (destructive) end of the spectrum. An adequate protein intake becomes even more important for women over the age of 40 who want to hold onto the lean muscle mass that is typically lost with age.

But keep in mind that there is an upper limit to how much protein the body can actually use.

If protein is so fundamentally important, it seems logical to think that more is better. But this simply isn't the case. Dietary proteins are the most energy-intensive macronutrient to digest and utilize. And their breakdown results in nitrogenous wastes (like ammonia and urea) that the liver and kidneys have to work overtime to process and excrete (through sweat and urine).

Just as there are negative consequences to consuming too many carbohydrates, there are some very real downsides to eating too much protein.

Eating more protein than your body needs can interfere with your health, performance, and recovery goals in a number of different ways. Weight gain, excess body fat, kidney stress, bone mineral imbalances, and dehydration are all the result of eating too much protein.

While there are no strict protein intake rules to follow, there are a few general guidelines. In addition to maintaining a focus on quality versus quantity, remember to slow down and enjoy what you're eating. Taking the time to chew your food will make it more satiating because the body's ability to extract and utilize what your body wants most from any protein source—its essential amino acids—will improve.

When animal proteins are on the menu, consider the use of a digestive enzyme supplement that contains betaine hydrochloride to further support the efficiency of your digestive process.

Is Animal Protein Necessary?

The consumption of animal protein is a sensitive topic on many levels. From a purely scientific standpoint, the evidence weighs heavily in its favor. When compared gram for gram, studies confirm that animal proteins are more easily and fully utilized than plant proteins. This makes sense given what we know about their biological value. Animal proteins contain not only a greater number but a better balance of the eight essential amino acids.

From an evolutionary standpoint, there's some fairly conclusive evidence to support the idea that animal protein was a foundational component of the human diet. Isotope analysis from archaeological studies suggests that our hominid ancestors began eating meat at least 2.5 million years ago. While the digestive process of our even more primitive relatives (the chimpanzees) was dominated by the large intestine (which is good for breaking down fiber, seeds, and other hard-to-digest plant foods), modern humans have a larger small intestine, which suggests that we have adapted to eating more digestible, bioavailable, and energy-dense foods (like meat).

When evaluated in terms of sheer nutrient density, animal protein sources such as beef, lamb, pork, poultry, and fish all have an essential amino acid profile that is far superior to that of any plant. In the simplest and clearest of terms, animal proteins are complete, plant proteins are not.

Meat also tends to be high in several key nutrients that are often lacking in plants. Leading the list are **iron** and **zinc** which, ironically, are the two most commonly cited nutrient deficiencies among both male and female athletes. The heme iron (found only in animals) is a particularly important mineral for menstruating women, and it's much more readily absorbed than the non-heme form found in plants. Zinc is difficult to source from plants, but it's abundant in beef, pork, and lamb. It's also better absorbed and utilized when it comes from an animal.

Vitamin B12 is another key nutrient for optimal health, performance, and recovery that cannot be found in any plant. **Docosahexaenoic acid or DHA** is an essential omega-3 fat that's abundant in fatty fish, but very difficult to obtain from plants. Other important nutrients found only in animal protein include:

CoenzymeQ10 (CoQ10), which is essential for the production of cellular energy. Our neurological, muscular, and cardiovascular function all rely on an adequate supply of CoQ10. It's also a powerful antioxidant.

Carnosine is another antioxidant that's concentrated in the muscles and brain. It contributes to improved muscular endurance.

Creatine is an important cellular energy molecule that's also stored in muscles and concentrated in the brain. Creatine functions as an easily accessible energy reserve for muscle cells, increasing their strength and endurance.

Of course there are many nutrients found in plants that can't be found in animals. So the best course of action is to eat an adequate and balanced amount of both in order to nourish your body as deeply and broadly as possible.

Keep in mind that we evolved eating the entire animal, not just its flesh as the vast majority (of Americans) do today. Animal flesh does contain an inflammatory amino acid called methionine which needs to be counterbalanced by the anti-inflammatory **glycine** and **proline**. These amino acids are found in the tendons, ligaments, and organs of animals, so their intake probably isn't in your culinary comfort zone. I know it's not in mine.

Luckily, several palatable and relatively inexpensive alternatives exist. You can sip some bone broth, mix up a batch of gelatin blocks, or blend a scoop of grass-fed collagen into a smoothie in order to boost your body's glycine and proline levels. Pre-packaged bone broths are available at any natural food store, although it's not that difficult to make your own. See page 115 for a recipe.

GET BACK IN THE GAME

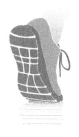

Obstacle Two

Macronutrient Imbalances

In Chapter One we discussed the unreliability of calorie counting as a method for assessing and tracking the body's need for energy. In addition to being inaccurate, it only allows for measuring the quantity (number of calories) not the quality (nutrient density) of the foods we eat. Portion control guidelines (like eating a tablespoon of fat or fist-sized serving of protein) offer a somewhat improved approach to deciding how much of what we should be eating. But continually counting, measuring, and otherwise micro-managing meals won't serve as a sane or sustainable long-term solution for satisfying the body's unique nutrient needs.

We also took an in-depth look at the structure and function of carbohydrates, fats, and proteins—the three, essential macronutrients the body uses to create energy. In this chapter we'll focus on fine-tuning macronutrient intake for optimal female health, performance, and recovery.

Macronutrient Ratios Matter

When we eat a meal, our primary energy goal is to provide the body with an adequate and balanced supply of all the raw materials it needs to stay fueled for several hours. In order to achieve this, it's necessary to consume the correct mix of macronutrients.

 Determining how many carbohydrates, fats, and proteins your body needs to thrive—not just survive—is essential for optimal health, performance, and recovery.

A woman's age, body composition, genetics, and training routine all influence her macronutrient metabolism. Some women can achieve their health, performance, and recovery goals by following a lower-carbohydrate, higher-fat diet. Others thrive on a few more carbohydrates and a little bit less fat. Almost all female athletes feel and perform better with at least a moderate amount of protein.

A woman's menstrual cycle will also create fluctuations in both her energy needs and metabolic processes over the course of any given month. As estrogen levels reach high and low points, the female body becomes a little more or a little less efficient at utilizing carbohydrates, fats, and proteins. So a female athlete's macronutrient goals can be a bit more of a moving target.

 Exploring the concept of fat adaptation—and the role it plays in determining a woman's ideal macronutrient mix—offers some important insights.

Fat adaptation is a metabolic state in which the body recognizes both dietary and stored fat as a readily accessible source of energy. The ability to mobilize and utilize stored fat for energy will reduce the body's dependence on glycogen (stored carbohydrates), which can be a huge benefit for endurance and ultra-endurance athletes. While many female athletes don't burn fat as a primary fuel source because they've become accustomed to following a higher carbohydrate diet, becoming fat-adapted offers many metabolic advantages.

As Mark Sisson, the bestselling author of The Primal Blueprint explains, "Fat adaptation is the normal, preferred metabolic state of the human animal. It's nothing special; it's just how we're meant to be."

Ultimately, fat adaption encourages metabolic flexibility; it allows the body to burn both fats and carbohydrates—effortlessly switching between the two fuel sources—depending on its specific needs. The fat-adapted athlete will be able to empty her glycogen stores through intense exercise, then refill them; move on to burning whatever dietary fat hasn't been stored, then easily access and utilize stored fat when that becomes necessary.

Many female athletes have found that following a paleolithic-type diet with its emphasis on eating what our hunter-gatherer ancestors ate (fewer carbohydrates, a moderate amount of protein, and an adequate supply of healthy fat) has made a significant and positive difference in how they look, feel, and perform. In addition to feeling less hungry and enjoying more consistent energy throughout the day, women may benefit most from its anti-inflammatory effects.

How do you know if your body is fat adapted? Ask yourself the following questions:

1. Does skipping a meal cause me to suffer from ravenous hunger, anxiety, headaches, and brain fog; or can I easily and comfortably go four to five hours without eating?
2. Do I experience peaks and valleys of energy that often leave me longing for a nap; or do I enjoy steady, even energy throughout the day?
3. Do I struggle to maintain a lean body composition; or am I relatively unconcerned about carrying excess body fat?
4. Do I need to eat something the minute I wake up; or can I do 30 to 45 minutes of low to medium intensity exercise in the morning before I eat?

If you answered "yes" to (the latter part of) all four of these questions, you have achieved a state of metabolic efficiency that allows for more effortless eating. You might get a little hungry, but you won't 'crash and burn' if you happen to miss a meal. You can access and burn stored body fat when you need to, without consuming any carbohydrates. When you do have an ample supply of glucose (blood sugar), your body will be able to use that without becoming dependent on it.

If you answered "no" to most of these questions, it might be time to evaluate the composition of your meals and re-balance your macronutrient intake.

How do you know what percentage of carbohydrates, fats, and proteins you should be eating?

There are as many answers to this question as there are female athletes. While it requires patience and perseverance, a fair amount of personal experimentation will be necessary. Begin by using a free app like *Cronometer* to keep a three or four-day food log in order to establish a baseline measurement of your current macronutrient intake totals before making any modifications.

As a very general recommendation, strive for a macronutrient balance that's 20 to 30% complex carbohydrates, 30 to 40% high-quality protein, and 30 to 40% healthy fat (based on caloric intake, not portion size). Establishing some initial macronutrient targets will give you a direction to move in and, eventually, determine the ratio that's right for you. If you begin to experience fewer food cravings or find that you're less hungry between meals, you're moving in the right direction.

The end goal is to learn how you need to fuel your body with lasting and consistent energy. When you achieve this goal, a lot of good things will begin to happen. From a metabolic standpoint, your blood sugar and insulin levels will remain low, keeping cortisol (a stress hormone) in check so you'll feel calmer and enjoy more even energy. Since your body's inflammatory and immune responses won't be activated or depleted, you might have fewer aches and pains and get sick less often. If you do get injured or become ill, you may find that you 'bounce back' quicker since all your energy resources can be fully mobilized and utilized for positive, productive, and regenerative purposes. Maintaining a lean body composition, regardless of your activity level, will probably require less attention and effort, too.

Feel good about sticking to the diet that works for you, regardless of what philosophy it resembles—low-carbohydrate, high-protein, low-fat, high-fat; Mediterranean, paleo, keto, or vegetarian. In many cases, these dietary schools of thought revolve around the central objective of weight loss. But the pursuit of optimal health, performance, and recovery is the bigger-picture priority.

As you begin to create a long-term plan for optimizing your macronutrient balance, establish some measurable criteria for tracking your progress.

Here's a short list of a few variables you might want to follow. Are you:

- Falling asleep any easier?
- Sleeping more soundly?
- Feeling calmer?
- Having an easier time with digestion and elimination?
- Becoming more motivated to set goals and start new projects?
- Able to go four to five hours between meals without feeling hungry and/or experiencing changes in your energy, mood, or ability to concentrate?

Pick the parameters that are most relevant and meaningful to you, and make sure that they are measurable. Write down the number of times you wake at night, for example; or assess your energy or irritability on a scale from one to five. Allow your body a week or two to adapt to any major macronutrient changes before you make further adjustments.

You may also want to consider opening a free *FitDay* account so you can have a more organized tracking system in place. Don't let it become a time-consuming chore; invest a few minutes for two or three days before you start making any macronutrient modifications so you can get a quantifiable sense of what your current ratios of fats, proteins, and carbohydrates are. Repeat the process again after you feel like you've made some significant changes.

Adjusting Your Carbohydrate Intake

Although conventional wisdom suggests that women should eat more carbohydrates than men, recent research confirms the female body's natural preference for fat as fuel. Several studies have shown that women derive more energy from fats and men more energy from carbohydrates while exercising. Even at rest, women burn more fat than men.

Female athletes still need to eat carbohydrates—sometimes in very different amounts. A soccer player's carbohydrate requirements will be completely different from those of an ultra-distance swimmer. Because a woman's ability to efficiently convert glycogen to energy declines with age, the 25 and 65-year-old 5K running specialists will also have very different carbohydrate needs. If a triathlete was actively training for a Half Ironman but suffered an injury that made it impossible for her to run and limited her time on the bike, her need for carbohydrates will be significantly reduced. An athlete's personal circumstances must always be taken into account.

 Since every female athlete is biologically unique, the beneficial (or detrimental) effects of carbohydrates will vary regardless of her chosen sport or activity level.

Discovering what works for you (a one-of-a-kind woman) will lead to maximum health and performance gains. Determining your carbohydrate 'sweet spot' will allow you to fine-tune your engine's fuel.

Very active athletes will likely feel and perform better with more carbohydrates since their energy demands will be higher than those of more sedentary women. But they should still avoid consuming more than what's necessary. The more glucose the body has to process, the more rapidly its cells are required to replicate or divide. Since cells are programmed to divide only a certain number of times, it becomes important to minimize their replacement rate. The more frequently our cells are replaced, the more rapidly our bodies age. In the case of carbohydrates, less can be more.

You may want to consider eating fewer carbohydrates if:

You 'bonk' frequently or need a constant supply of carbohydrate-based fuels to get you through training and competition. If you can't do 30 to 45 minutes of low to medium intensity exercise in the morning before eating without feeling light headed or you're often left physically and mentally fatigued from an hour or less of moderate exercise during the day, your health and performance may both benefit from becoming less reliant on the inherently small carbohydrate storage capacity of the body.

You have sugar cravings. Pay particular attention to what you're eating for breakfast. Is it a bowl of instant oatmeal with fruit and sugar? A breakfast that doesn't contain protein and/or fat may set you up for an early morning ride on the blood sugar roller coaster—and for a battle with sugar cravings all day. Focus on eating protein and fat for breakfast, shifting your intake of carbohydrates to later in the day or after exercise. Several research studies have shown that women who follow a low-carbohydrate diet have fewer sugar cravings than those who follow a low-fat diet. If you're constantly craving sugar, reducing your carbohydrate intake might be helpful.

You're constantly hungry. The food we eat contains more than calories to satiate hunger; it provides the body with essential nutrients like fiber, protein, and fat. Simple, refined carbohydrates lack nutrients, even if they do (temporarily) fill us up and provide us with energy. No matter how many simple carbohydrates we eat, the body will still seek out the additional nutrients it needs. Adopting a strategy for eating higher-quality fuel in the form of proteins, fats, and a minimal to moderate amount of complex carbohydrates can provide your body with a slower-burning and longer-lasting source of energy.

You experience frequent gas and bloating. Eating too many carbohydrates can often lead to gas and bloating. If you eat lots of fruits, vegetables, grains, and beans, the problem might be too much fiber. Fiber is technically a type of carbohydrate that's not digestible, so it adds very few calories to your diet. Resistant starch is a type of dietary fiber that passes through the small intestine undigested, but can be used as a fuel source (prebiotic) by the beneficial bacteria living in the large intestine.

Some types of indigestible fiber classified as FODMAP's (fermentable oligo-di-monosaccharides and polyols) can be problematic, particularly for women who suffer from irritable bowel syndrome or IBS. Like resistant starches, FODMAPs fuel bacterial growth. They are more likely to create unpleasant digestive symptoms, however, because they are processed at a much slower rate.

Sometimes resistant starches are found in foods that are also high in FODMAPs. These foods include wheat-based pastas, rye bread, and white beans. Avoid these foods if you have IBS or are following a low FODMAP diet.

Fructose can also cause digestive difficulties for many women; those who are postmenopausal are most at risk. Fructose is a type of carbohydrate found mostly in fruit, dried fruit, and fruit-based sweeteners. Some women suffer from a fructose intolerance that causes gas and bloating. Lower fructose fruit choices include apricots, nectarines, peaches, cantaloupe, pineapple, raspberries, blackberries, strawberries, clementines, and grapefruit.

You have a family history of type 2 diabetes, high blood pressure, or heart disease. All carbohydrates are eventually broken down into glucose or sugar. The more you consume, the more insulin your pancreas produces. And the more likely you are to become insulin-resistant as the cells in your muscles, stored body fat, and liver eventually become exhausted from being forced to process excessive amounts of sugar. In order to protect the body from toxicity, insulin encourages the cells and systems of the body to accept as much glucose from the bloodstream as possible. Type 2 diabetes is the end result of this protective metabolic process calling it quits and shutting down.

In addition to preventing the onset of type 2 diabetes, eating fewer carbohydrates may be the key to a healthier heart. That's the finding from a ten-year, worldwide study of more than 125,000 people. In fact, consuming more dietary fat (about 35% of total calories in this case) was associated with a lower risk of heart disease and related death. A high-carbohydrate diet (more than 60% of total calories) was linked to a higher heart disease risk. According to the Centers for Disease Control and Prevention statistics, the average American adult gets close to 50% of their daily calories from carbohydrates.

 While eating fewer carbohydrates (and becoming fat adapted) can result in many health and performance benefits, consuming too few can be counterproductive.

When women don't consume enough carbohydrates their estradiol levels fall and estrone levels increase, triggering a fight or flight response. Estrone (a type of estrogen) is a pro-inflammatory female hormone created and secreted by fat cells. When the body exists in a chronic state of increased inflammation (and stress), it begins to store as much fat as possible in order to prepare and protect itself from an impending (although imaginary) emergency—such as a food shortage.

There may be times when you need to consider eating more carbohydrates, even if you are a fat-adapted athlete. These include:

You tire easily when you really shouldn't. If you find that you're frequently tired, completely out of energy by the end of the day, or out of breath after climbing a flight or two of stairs despite being moderately to very fit, you may need to increase your carbohydrate intake. Of course, iron deficiency is always on the table as the root cause of excessive or unexplained fatigue. Every woman—menstruating or not—should have their red blood cell count, serum iron, and ferritin iron levels checked at least once a year.

You frequently feel cold. A low-carbohydrate diet can cause hypothyroidism—or at least its symptoms. This is because the body needs an adequate supply of glucose to make the thyroid hormone T3 from its parent source, T4. T3 is the 'free' or bioactive form of thyroid hormone that actually delivers energy (and therefore heat) to the cells. Feeling cold is a common symptom of hypothyroidism or a functional thyroid weakness.

You lead a high-stress life. Carbohydrates are necessary for supporting the health of the adrenal glands. In the absence of an adequate supply of the easily utilized energy that comes from carbohydrates, the adrenal glands have to work harder at maintaining adequate glucose levels in the blood. When they are forced to work harder, the adrenal glands increase their production of the stress hormone cortisol. Erratic and recurring cortisol spikes are a major contributor to the onset of adrenal fatigue.

An adequate supply of carbohydrates is also necessary for the production of serotonin. Serotonin is the calming, 'feel-good' neurotransmitter that can enhance a woman's overall sense of wellbeing. So an adequate—but not excessive—carbohydrate intake might help you feel more relaxed, even during periods of increased stress.

You don't sleep well. In addition to its calming effects, serotonin helps women sleep more soundly. A meal that includes about 20 grams of a complex carbohydrate (like sweet potato) three to four hours before bed has been shown to measurably improve sleep quality.

You have irregular, absent, or painful menstrual cycles. Sometimes a woman experiences menstrual irregularities because her 'primitive brain' has convinced her body to become less fertile in an effort to prepare and protect itself from some imminent threat (like a famine). To function optimally, the female body needs to be satiated in order to feel safe. Consuming the appropriate amount of the right kind of carbohydrates can encourage the body to remain balanced, knowing that it's macronutrient needs are being met.

Choose Complex Carbohydrates First

Carbohydrates are constructed of three simple components—sugar, fiber, and starch. Simple carbohydrates are sugar; they are devoid of any other nutrients, require little digestion, and are absorbed very quickly into the bloodstream. While there is a time and a place for these to be used (typically before, during, and/or after athletic events), complex carbohydrates are a better day-to-day choice because they contain more nutrients. Since they are higher in fiber, they digest and release their energy more slowly. This not only makes them more satiating, but much less likely to create harmful blood sugar spikes.

In addition to being packed with more nutrients, complex carbohydrates offer a fuller range of flavors to enjoy. When food shopping, use the chart below as a quick reference guide. Because root vegetables are lower in simple sugars and don't contain anti-nutrients (nutrients that interfere with the absorption and utilization of other nutrients), they should always be a first choice.

The Best Sources of Complex Carbohydrates

Root Vegetables

Sweet potatoes and yams	Parsnips
Winter squashes	Turnips
Butternut squash	Jerusalem artichokes
Heirloom potatoes	Carrots
Beets	Rutabaga

Fruits

Berries	Grapefruit
Watermelon and cantaloupe	Mango
Papaya	Guava
Apple	Fresh figs
Tangerines and oranges	Slightly green bananas
	Plantains

Beans

- Black Beans
- Black-eyed peas
- Chickpeas
- Great northern beans
- Kidney beans
- Lentils
- Lima beans
- Navy beans
- Pinto beans
- Split peas

Grains

- Quinoa
- Wild rice
- Steel cut oats
- Millet
- Buckwheat
- Amaranth
- Teff
- Rye
- Emmer and einkorn wheat
- Sorghum

What's Wrong with Rice?

While (white) rice is often considered a good source of easily-digestible glucose (sugar) that is sometimes even endorsed by primal diet enthusiasts because it can be transformed into a source of resistant starch (fuel for the beneficial bacteria living in the large intestine) when cooked and cooled, it contains arsenic.

As known carcinogen, arsenic in rice has been a concern since a 2012 study conducted by *Consumer Reports* found high levels of this toxic heavy metal in various brands of rice products. According to the U.S. Food and Drug Administration, "Rice has higher levels of arsenic than other foods, in part because as rice plants grow, the plant and grain tend to absorb arsenic more readily than other food crops."

In fact, rice has 10 to 20 times more arsenic than other cereal crops because it is grown in flooded fields, an environment that encourages arsenic absorption. Some types of rice do have less arsenic than others. This is a brief synopsis of what we currently know:

- Basmati rice is lower in arsenic than any other kind of rice.
- Brown rice contains more arsenic than white rice because it's concentrated in the husk. In addition to storing more toxins, the hard outer shells of all grains can irritate the digestive tract. They also contain anti-nutrients that bind to vitamins and minerals, preventing their absorption.
- Levels of arsenic are the same in organically and conventionally grown rice.
- Rice cakes and crackers can contain arsenic levels higher than those in cooked rice.
- The levels of arsenic found in rice milk are significantly more than what's legally allowed in drinking water.

The *Consumer Reports* study (referenced above) found California basmati rice to be the least contaminated of all varieties evaluated. Lundberg Family Farms (a California company) is my go-to brand because they safety test their rice. According to published results, the company's 2016 crop registered 0.090 parts per million of arsenic, slightly below its previous six-year average of 0.093.

To reduce your arsenic exposure, rotate the grains you eat. Farro, barley, and quinoa contain significantly less arsenic than rice; amaranth, buckwheat, millet and polenta have virtually none.

To remove the most arsenic from your rice:

1. Soak it overnight. This will open up the grain, allowing the arsenic to escape.
2. Drain the rice and rinse it thoroughly with fresh water.
3. For every part rice, add 5 parts water and cook the rice until tender. Do not allow it to absorb all the water (boil dry).
4. Drain the rice and rinse it again with hot water in order to get rid of any arsenic remnants left in the cooking water.

The Case Against Carbohydrate Cycling

Carbohydrate cycling involves making planned adjustments to your daily carbohydrate intake in an effort to prevent or overcome a fat loss or performance plateau. While there isn't a standard protocol, one typical approach includes the implementation of lower and higher-carbohydrate days. Fat intake increases on lower-carbohydrate days and decreases on higher-carbohydrate days while protein intake remains the same. The other common approach involves keeping both protein and fat intake fairly consistent, modifying only carbohydrate intake on certain days of the week. With this method, lower-carbohydrate days also become lower-calorie days.

Proponents claim that carbohydrate cycling can help increase muscle mass, decrease body fat, and improve athletic performance. But female-specific research on the subject is limited; the overwhelming majority has been done on men.

While some evidence suggests that brief and relatively infrequent periods of carbohydrate restriction (and fasting) can result in short-term metabolic benefits, carbohydrate cycling should not be viewed as a viable, long-term solution for achieving your health, performance and/or body composition goals. In fact, women can be adversely affected by this dietary practice for a number of reasons.

Women are, in general, more sensitive to the effects of carbohydrates than men. And prolonged or repetitive macronutrient restriction has been shown to interfere with female metabolism and thyroid hormone production. The female hormones estrogen and progesterone can also influence a woman's ability to utilize carbohydrates. At different points in the menstrual cycle, carbohydrates are either processed a little more readily (during the first half) or with a little more difficulty (during the second half), making them a little more likely to be stored as fat. Because male hormone levels aren't as easily influenced and don't regularly fluctuate, carbohydrate cycling may be more beneficial for men.

Adjusting Your Fat Intake

Our understanding of dietary fats has evolved over the past few decades. For many years, scientists told us that too much saturated fat (commonly found in animal products, coconut, and palm oils) was bad for our hearts; they advised us to switch to plant-based polyunsaturated fats instead. But research has definitively discredited the misguided notion that saturated fats are harmful. They are an excellent source of slow-burning energy that support healthy hormonal, nervous, metabolic, and cellular function—when eaten in the right amount.

While some polyunsaturated fats do offer health benefits, they should be consumed with caution. Processed vegetable oils (like canola, corn, soybean, sunflower, and safflower) are high in omega-6 fatty acids and considered pro-inflammatory. These fats act as hormone and immune function disruptors. However, monounsaturated fats (found in macadamia nuts, avocados, and olives) are universally accepted as healthy. These fats enhance cellular, cardiovascular, and immune function.

 As a general guideline, healthy fats can be found in fresh, whole, and unprocessed foods; the unhealthy in those that are refined, processed, and packaged.

As a very general recommendation, focus on achieving a balanced intake of dietary fats with a third of them coming from saturates, a third from monounsaturates, and a third from the polyunsaturates that are high in omega 3's (primarily fish and fish oil supplements).

How much total fat should you be eating? It depends on many different variables including your genetics, metabolism, hormonal status, training regimen, and diet.

There are times to consider eating more fat. These include:

You're constantly hungry. Fat not only makes food taste good, it satiates hunger. Healthy fats are the best source of long, slow, and clean burning energy for the body, so it's a clear case of 'nature knows best.' Fatty, grass-fed meat cuts offer both saturated and monounsaturated fats, along with a serving of high-quality protein. Avocados, cheese, yogurt, whole eggs, fish (especially salmon and trout), and nuts (especially almonds, Brazil nuts, hazelnuts, pecans, pistachios, and macadamias) are some other high-fat foods that are both delicious and nutritious.

Your joints ache. Joints can feel achy for many different reasons. The root cause might be poor mobility or improper movement mechanics; weak or tight muscles. Regardless of the reason, addressing and minimizing chronic inflammation can help reduce the pain. Consuming more omega-3 fats is a sound, anti-inflammatory strategy to implement.

You have difficulty losing weight. Medical research has proven that adhering to a low-fat diet will slow a woman's metabolism down. And eating larger amounts of carbohydrate calories in place of fat calories can result in a number of health and performance-draining problems including stubborn weight loss, type 2 diabetes, high triglyceride levels, and poor cognitive function.

Your physical performance and/or recovery is lagging. Fat, specifically saturated fat, plays a key role in supporting optimal physical performance. In fact, the female body can't make an adequate supply of the strength and recovery hormones (DHEA and testosterone) it needs without it.

You find it difficult to remain focused. If you frequently feel like your mind is foggy or you just can't concentrate, you might need to eat more fat. While the brain prefers glucose as its primary form of fuel, a number of studies show that eating specific fatty acids (like the medium chain triglycerides found in coconut oil) can improve brain function by increasing ketones—a form of clean-burning energy.

You have fertility issues. Fat intake is crucial for keeping your hormones balanced which, in turn, helps keep your reproductive system healthy. Both men and women use dietary fat to make sex hormones like estrogen and testosterone. In extreme cases, a lack of dietary fat can cause infertility.

You have dry skin and hair. Sebum is the body's natural moisturizer and we have no problem producing it as long as we have enough fatty acids available. Some of these fats can be created by the body while others need to come from food. If dry skin and hair are an issue for you, eating a wide variety of healthy saturated and unsaturated fats can help. While unsaturated fats (like olive oil) are important for preventing dry skin, saturated fats (like coconut oil) are necessary, too. Both types of fats are used to build new skin cells and keep the existing skin supple. Hair gets most of its support from vitamins, many of which are fat-soluble. Eating more fat will allow your hair to more fully absorb these nutrients.

 With all the benefits fat provides, it might seem that more is better. But remember: it's all about recognizing and satisfying your body's unique macronutrient needs.

While some women may thrive eating more healthy fat, others will look, feel, and perform better with less.

There are times to consider reducing your fat intake. These include:

You're not eating healthy fat. Processed, refined fats are possibly the most harmful food-like substance we can eat. Not only do they cause oxidative stress (when harmful free radicals outnumber helpful antioxidants and begin to damage healthy cells and tissues), they are actively incorporated into the body's cellular membranes causing inflammatory disease and metabolic dysfunction. Maintaining healthy cell membranes is critically important because they act as gatekeepers; they allow nutrients to enter and waste products to exit the cell. Due to their unnatural rigidity, refined fats make the cell membranes less pliable and permeable, diminishing the function of the cell and the health of the body.

Your total intake of healthy fats is exceeding your body's energy demands. In other words, when excess fat calories are causing you to gain weight. Healthy fats can support an increase in lean body mass. So it's important to determine if the weight gain is coming from new muscle or extra fat. The occasional assessment of your body fat percentage is the most objective way to measure and monitor your body composition.

Lab tests indicate that your lipids (total cholesterol and low density lipoproteins) have increased. Although we now know that cholesterol is not a cardiovascular villain, seeing it rise rapidly (by 25% or more) is an indicator that your body may not be able to utilize large amounts of saturated, dietary fats. While a *Bulletproof*™ coffee every morning may serve as a tasty and satisfying source of slow-burning energy for some women, its heavy fat content can have negative consequences for others.

The inflammatory symptoms that initially disappeared by increasing your healthy fat intake reappear. The omega-3 and omega-6 fats are used by the body to create hormone-like chemicals called *prostaglandins*. Prostaglandins are a group of physiologically active fat compounds that are found in almost every human tissue. They manage and influence a wide range of metabolic processes which include the regulation of pain and inflammation.

As is the case with many hormones, prostaglandins can play a necessary yet opposing role in the body. They are the reason we develop a fever in response to a viral infection or develop swelling after an injury. NSAIDs (non-steroidal anti-inflammatory drugs) like ibuprofen and aspirin are used to block the effects of the prostaglandins that cause fever, pain, and swelling.

An increase in prostaglandins can be beneficial in acute or short-term circumstances, but they can be detrimental when chronically elevated. While eating more healthy fats might initially improve an inflammatory condition (like joint pain), the presenting symptoms can return, over time, due to an over-corrected (and therefore inflammatory) fat intake.

The Ketogenic Diet for Females

The ketogenic (keto) diet is a very low-carbohydrate, high-fat diet that promotes the metabolic formation of ketone bodies (made by the liver from fatty acids during periods of low food intake), which prompt the body to use fat as its primary energy source. The keto diet (a variation of the old Atkins diet) is becoming more widely embraced for its numerous health benefits which include weight loss and improved blood sugar, cholesterol, and triglyceride levels. In fact, the ketogenic diet can prevent and reverse metabolic syndrome, a collection of symptoms that all contribute to the onset of obesity, diabetes, high blood pressure, and heart disease.

Following a keto diet requires entering a fasted state in order to 'teach' the body how to access and burn both dietary and stored body fat as its principal source of fuel. Fasting is considered a hormetic stressor—a stressful input (no food) that encourages an adaptive response (like fat loss). Experiencing some hormetic stress can be very beneficial; feeling a little hungry, a little too hot, or a little too cold from time to time is okay. In fact, it can make us stronger and healthier. But when a hormetic stress is too large, it transforms into a more generalized and harmful form of stress.

The size of any hormetic stress is, of course, relative. What's hormetic for you might be overly stressful for me. Many different variables affect how much of any given hormetic stressor an individual can tolerate. In general, women have a much lower hormetic stress threshold than men.

Fasting is essentially planned, simulated starvation. And to be beneficial, intermittent fasting (a foundational component of the ketogenic diet) needs to be done regularly. The specifics can vary. 'Fasting' might mean waiting to eat breakfast until you feel hungry (a sound and sustainable strategy). Or it might involve avoiding food for an entire day once a week, once a month or even for multiple, back-to-back days a few times a year. Unfortunately, the vast majority of studies that confirm the benefits of repetitive, long-term fasting have been done on men; there is little information available on how this process of planned deprivation specifically affects women.

In one of the few studies done on women, researchers found that a two-day fast shifted nervous system activity toward sympathetic (fight or flight) dominance. While their cognitive abilities remained unaffected, the fasting women felt anxious and stressed. In men, a two-day fast shifted nervous system dominance in the opposite direction—toward parasympathetic (rest and digest) dominance. They reported feeling well-rested and relaxed; their blood pressure decreased and cognitive abilities increased.

In addition to fat loss, one of the main benefits of intermittent fasting is increased autophagy (self-digestion), which improves the body's ability to utilize old and/or damaged cells for the energy it needs to create new ones. The results of research done on intermittent fasting and autophagy, however, have revealed a significant difference between the way men and women respond. While one study showed that male neurons responded to starvation by undergoing autophagy, female neurons respond by resisting autophagy.

At the end of the day, biology will strive to protect a woman's ability to reproduce. So women will be inherently more prone to having a negative response to any energy deficit. Even if you don't have an interest in becoming pregnant, the status of your fertility (which is influenced by how broadly and deeply your body is nourished) plays a pivotal role in determining the status of your overall health.

Based on the limited research that exists, it appears that menopausal and postmenopausal women are less likely to benefit from intermittent fasting or a ketogenic diet than men. There do appear to be some solid therapeutic benefits for those who are undergoing chemotherapy and/or being treated for age-related neurodegeneration. Few conclusions have been drawn about the diet's effects on younger women.

The bottom line, at least for now? Women are less likely to benefit from following a long-term ketogenic diet than men. There may, however, be a place for shorter fasts in the interest of promoting autophagy. If you're in the habit of constantly eating or 'grazing' throughout the day, your cells won't have a chance to repair or rid themselves of the wastes and toxins they have accumulated. Short periods of fasting can give them an opportunity to take care of those tasks.

Remember that fasting and/or following a ketogenic diet will limit your total intake of certain nutrients. So entering and maintaining ketosis for prolonged periods of time may not be beneficial unless you have a good reason—you are obese and have a significant amount of body fat to lose, have an autoimmune disease, are diabetic, undergoing some form of cancer treatment, or receiving therapy for cognitive decline or dementia.

Adjusting Your Protein Intake

While people tend to disagree more about the relative importance of fats versus carbohydrates in the ongoing energy debate, almost everyone—especially athletes—can agree on the foundational importance of protein.

Muscles are largely made of protein. And as with most tissues in the body, they are constantly being broken down and rebuilt. To gain muscle, your body must synthesize (use) more protein than it breaks down. So a higher protein will naturally support the body's ability to build and maintain muscle. Even if your training goals don't include the addition of muscular mass, you are a physically active woman. And physically active women need more protein.

Female athletes over the age of 40 will also need more protein. Those who are in the initial stages of recovering from a serious illness or activity-interrupting injury will need less protein than when actively training, but more than what's required to support their BMR (basal metabolic rate). At a minimum, active women should be taking in about one gram of protein for each pound of their body weight daily. Although it is universally agreed that protein is an essential component of a complete and nourishing diet, many female athletes simply don't eat enough of it.

These red flags may be a warning that your protein intake is too low:

You're constantly hungry. Under normal circumstances, eating protein reduces ghrelin, the body's hunger hormone. It also triggers the release of the body's satiety hormone (peptide YY), which makes you feel full. The satiating effects of dietary protein can be powerful. In fact, one study showed that increasing protein from 15 to 30% of the total calories consumed by a group of overweight women led to their eating 441 fewer calories a day—without any planned or intentional restriction of their food intake.

You have difficulty building or maintaining muscle mass. Numerous studies show that eating an adequate amount of protein can help build and maintain muscular size and strength. Keeping your protein intake high can also help prevent muscle loss when your body is in a catabolic (destructive) state—during periods of intense training, emotional stress, injury, or illness.

You are a postmenopausal woman concerned about bone health. Have you heard the myth that protein (especially animal protein) is bad for your bones? It's based on the idea that protein increases acidity in the body which, in turn, causes calcium (an alkalinizing agent) to be leached from the bones. It's important to note, however, that bones are mostly made of collagen—an animal-based protein. Most long-term studies confirm that dietary proteins offer major bone health benefits (when they are not eaten in excess). In fact, women who eat more protein tend to maintain their bone mass better as they get older, and they tend to have a much lower risk of both osteoporosis and bone fractures.

Your health, performance, and recovery goals include weight loss. We know that protein has a much higher thermic (heat-producing) effect than either fat or carbohydrates and researchers from Laval University have confirmed that a higher protein intake can measurably increase female metabolism. In fact, one of their studies found that a high-protein intake group of women burned 260 more calories per day than a low-protein group, with no difference in their levels of physical activity.

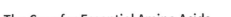

The Case for Essential Amino Acids

Essential amino acids (EAAs) are the basic building blocks of strength, energy, and recovery that our bodies have been programmed to extract from the dietary proteins we eat. In a very real and practical sense, athletes don't need more protein, they need more essential amino acids.

Without an adequate supply of essential amino acids, the body can't perform or recover well. Almost everyone—regardless of their age, gender, or activity level—can benefit from maintaining high and balanced serum levels of the essential amino acids responsible for strength, growth, and repair.

If you have your sights set on making strength or endurance gains, improving your body composition, or recovering faster and more completely from an injury or illness, consider the use of a high-quality EAA supplement that contains all eight of the essential amino acids, not just the three branched-chain (leucine, isoleucine, and valine). While there are proven muscular recovery benefits associated with the use of branched-chain amino acids (BCAAs), they do not provide the full and necessary spectrum of additional essential amino acids the body needs for its most immediate and pressing needs.

Think of the BCAAs as a small group of construction site managers whose job it is to plan and direct the future activity of a separate group of workers who are never present in the same place at the same time. EAAs, on the other hand, are a cohesive team of management and labor who show up together, working side-by-side, to complete a project.

A properly balanced EAA formula will contain the correct amino acid ratios and have a NNU of 99%. Because EAAs don't require any digestion, they won't create any metabolic (nitrogen) waste and will be rapidly absorbed (within 20 minutes) by the body for (almost) immediate use. Compare that to the three or four hours it takes the essential amino acids derived from dietary proteins to make their way into the bloodstream. Protein powders will be more quickly digested and easily assimilated than other dietary proteins. But a balanced essential amino acid product will be utilized five times more effectively for anabolic (strength and recovery) purposes.

Finding a properly formulated EAA formula that tastes good and doesn't contain any fillers, artificial flavors, or other objectionable ingredients can be difficult. The product I can personally recommend is *FundAminos*™. A single, five-gram serving of this high-quality, powdered product contains only four calories but provides the equivalent of 20 grams of dietary protein (about three ounces of lean meat). It's available on Amazon or at purecleanperformance.com.

Although women rarely eat too much protein, there are times you may want to consider eating less. These include:

You regularly experience meat sweats. Each type of macronutrient is digested and absorbed differently by the body. Carbohydrates are broken down quickly and easily, which means they don't require a lot of energy for processing. Proteins are much more complex; they take 20-30 times more energy to digest. As a result, they have a much higher thermic effect. The more protein you eat, the more energy the body expends. Eating excessive amounts of protein generates so much heat that the body has to sweat in order to cool itself down.

You're constantly thirsty. When your protein intake is too high, your kidneys are required to work overtime, flushing nitrogenous waste products out of the body through more frequent urination. This can significantly increase your body's need for fluids and, of course, your level of thirst.

You have a family history of kidney disease. According to a study published in *Nutrition and Metabolism*, adhering to a high-protein diet for an extended period of time might increase your risk of kidney disease. And eating too much protein can negatively affect those who suffer from an existing kidney condition. If you have a genetic predisposition for kidney-related issues, keep this information in mind. But remember that the two main risk factors for kidney failure are high blood pressure and diabetes. Research indicates that a higher protein intake can prevent both.

The Merits of Protein Cycling

The concept of protein cycling has been generating quite a bit of interest lately and its potential benefits are worth exploring. In order to discuss protein cycling, it's first necessary to understand protein sparing—the process by which the body derives energy from sources other than protein. These sources can include fatty tissues, dietary fats, glycogen, and carbohydrates. Since protein sparing preserves muscle tissue, protein cycling may be of particular value to women over the age of 40.

The practice of protein cycling is similar to that of intermittent fasting—shifting between periods of restricted and unrestricted macronutrient intake. Intermittent fasting activates autophagy when cells are given the opportunity to repair themselves and/or rid themselves of the wastes and toxins they have accumulated. Autophagy also stimulates the release of growth hormone, which boosts the body's ability to repair and regenerate.

Protein cycling involves alternating between periods of low protein consumption and normal to high protein consumption. Undereating protein on certain days of the week lowers insulin and raises glucagon—a hormone that stimulates and supports the body's ability to utilize both glucose and fats for energy. Higher levels of glucagon also activate autophagy.

Since the body can't make its own supply of protein, a scarcity will force it to become creative and recycle any unused, pre-existing proteins that may be available. This innately programmed recycling system encourages the body to identify and utilize its old or impaired cellular materials as a second-hand source of protein.

When it comes to protein cycling, a little can go a long way; you don't need to be in a constant state of protein deprivation in order to get results. In fact, many proponents suggest that benefits can be gained by implementing just one low-protein (fewer than 15 grams) day a week. Using a program like *Cronometer* for tracking purposes can make it easier.

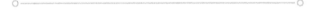

How to Make Your Own Protein Bars

Why make your own protein bars when there are dozens of different pre-made brands to choose from? Finding a high-quality bar with minimal ingredients and a well-balanced mix of macronutrients at a reasonable price isn't easy.

You don't need to spend lots of money on expensive, pre-packaged bars when you can easily make your own with a few simple ingredients that you probably already have at home.

This DIY recipe requires just five ingredients and takes about five minutes to make. As an added bonus, these tasty, well-balanced, and hunger-satisfying bars don't require any refrigeration so they can go where you go.

Ingredients:

- 2 cups (16 ounces) unsweetened almond butter (or the nut butter of your choice)
- ⅓ cup Lakanto (monk fruit-sweetened) maple syrup ⅓ cup coconut flour
- 1 ¼ cup Jarrow pumpkin seed protein powder
- ½ cup Lily's stevia-sweetened chocolate chips (optional)

Instructions:

1. Line an 8x8 or 8x10 inch pan with parchment paper and set aside.
2. In a large mixing bowl, add your dry ingredients and set aside.
3. Melt your nut butter with your sweetener on a stovetop, mixing until combined.
4. Combine your wet and dry ingredients to make a thick batter. Adjust your mixture with a little additional sweetener, coconut flour, or nut butter to suit your preferred taste and texture.
5. Transfer the batter to the lined pan and press firmly in place. Refrigerate.
6. Once firm, cut your nourishing creation into bite-size squares or larger bars.
7. Melt the (optional) chocolate chips; pour evenly over the squares or bars. Refrigerate until firm. The chocolate layer may require a second cut. Store in a glass, air-tight container.

Notes:

Pure maple syrup or raw honey can be substituted for the monk fruit syrup. These bars can be kept refrigerated (during warmer months) or frozen for longer storage.

There are endless variations to try: add some vanilla, almond, or pistachio extract; mix in some chopped nuts or (unmelted) chocolate chips; swap collagen powder for the protein powder, hazelnut or almond flour for the coconut flour, your favorite protein for the pumpkin seed powder.

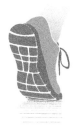

Obstacle Three

Poor Cellular Health

The human body contains trillions of different cells working constantly together to complete hundreds of specialized tasks. While we're not consciously aware of what's happening inside our bodies at the cellular level, there's a lot going on. Energy is always being made, waste products are continuously being cleared. Old cells are being replaced by news cells, which serve as the tiny building blocks of every tissue and organ system in the body.

 Optimal health, performance, and recovery all begin with good cellular health.

In Chapter Two we discussed the body's basic macronutrient requirements, and why eating the proper balance of macronutrients is an essential first step in providing for the body's cellular needs. **But cells have their own set of additional and very specific requirements which include:**

1. **An adequate supply of oxygen,** which is necessary for cellular respiration (energy production).
2. **Water,** which provides them with a transport system for delivering nutrients and getting rid of the waste products they inevitably generate.
3. **Micronutrients,** including vitamins and minerals, which are necessary for normal metabolic, enzymatic, and physiologic function.
4. **Antioxidants** to protect themselves from the damaging effects of oxidation (the harmful but unavoidable interaction between oxygen and living tissue).
5. **A clean environment** to live and work in. Because toxins are such an important issue, a full chapter of this book will be dedicated to discussing them.

Cellular Requirement #1: Oxygenation

In a healthy environment, cells have access to an extensive supply of oxygen and they can be repaired and rejuvenated by something as simple as a good night's sleep. Proper cellular oxygenation supports optimal energy production (cellular respiration), enhanced brain function, and an increased adaptation to both mental and physical stress. In many ways, the pursuit of optimal health, performance, and recovery are all dependent on sufficient cellular oxygenation.

When cells lack an adequate supply of oxygen, they struggle to produce energy, make mistakes when they replicate, and have a hard time cleaning themselves up once all their hard work is done. If the cells don't stay clean, the blood and other bodily fluids they live and work in become 'muddy' (which makes oxygen transport more difficult). Low oxygen (*hypoxemia*) is a primary cause of illness and disease; it weakens the immune system increasing the incidence of bacterial and viral infections, DNA mutations (which occur when a cell divides and doesn't copy itself correctly), systemic inflammation, delayed recovery, and premature aging.

What causes hypoxemia?

The most common cause of low oxygen is poor blood flow to the cells, which is typically attributed to a lack of fitness. While being 'out of shape' isn't a concern for most female athletes, other likely causes of hypoxemia include anemia, insufficient sleep, excessive physical and mental stress, prolonged exposure to toxins or electromagnetic fields (EMFs), and a low body pH (potential for hydrogen).

What can you do about it?

Plenty.

 Eating lots of acid-neutralizing, alkaline-rich foods like asparagus, avocados, broccoli, Brussels sprouts, cabbage, carrots, cauliflower, celery, collard greens, cucumbers, kale, lemons, limes, onions, spinach, seaweed, and watermelon can support cellular oxygenation.

A quick online search will yield a number of other high-alkaline food options, if these aren't practical or appealing.

There is a direct relationship between cellular oxygenation and the body's pH level. When the body becomes overly acidic, hydrogen begins to displace oxygen at the cellular level. This disrupts proper cellular function, leaving the body more susceptible to fatigue, injury, illness, and fragile bones (when the body is too acidic, it will steal calcium, potassium, and sodium from the bones to use as neutralizing agents). An acidic internal environment will also impair the body's ability to repair its damaged cells and tissues (including the muscles), and rid itself of toxins.

As the body's pH level increases (becomes more alkaline), the affinity (or bond) between oxygen and hemoglobin weakens. That means a larger supply of oxygen can be released and utilized by the cells and tissues. In fact, research indicates that alkaline tissues hold 20 times more oxygen than acidic tissues. In addition to eating more alkaline foods, take steps to minimize your intake of any acidifying, food-like substances that contain large amounts of artificial or refined sugars such as pre-packaged and processed foods, energy drinks, and soda.

Other simple strategies that can be used to improve the body's acid/alkaline balance include:

Using some simple baking soda. The alkalinizing and oxygenating effects of sodium bicarbonate were first documented by scientists in 1924, and they continue to be confirmed today. According to the American College of Sports Medicine, baking soda is still counted among the most commonly used ergogenic aids. Athletes use it to delay muscle fatigue and improve their overall physical performance through increased tissue oxygenation.

Sodium bicarbonate supplementation is especially useful during short bouts of high-intensity exercise. Sprinters, swimmers, and rowers have reported documented performance improvements when taking baking soda prior to competition. Recent research suggests that its use may also be beneficial during endurance-based training and racing events lasting 30 to 60 minutes.

During high-intensity workouts, the body releases chemicals that can be absorbed into muscle tissue when metabolic waste products (like lactic acid and hydrogen) are pushed into the muscle cells. While most of these performance-reducing chemicals are neutralized or eliminated, those that remain can rapidly establish an overly acidic environment. The use of baking soda prior to exercise creates a more favorable (alkaline) environment for the muscles, which allows them to clear metabolic wastes faster and more efficiently. This, in turn, improves performance while speeding recovery.

Bringing some awareness to the breath. Diaphragmatic breathing can increase your lung capacity, allowing you to take in more oxygen. When we breathe on 'autopilot' and exhale, a small amount of residual air is left behind in the lungs. Pulling the abdomen in slightly on the exhale engages the diaphragm and forces all the air out. A more active exhalation creates additional space for fresh, oxygenated air to enter the lungs on the next inhalation.

Practice diaphragmatic breathing by taking slow, relaxed, and even breaths. Allow your stomach to expand without any holding or restriction. Try to inhale for a count of six; hold for four, and exhale for six. Repeat this process six to eight times. With continued practice, diaphragmatic breathing will become more automatic. Completing a round of diaphragmatic breathing before each meal can help make your practice more routine. And it offers the added benefit of relaxing the nervous system, which improves digestion.

Taking some measurements. Women who want more tangible feedback could consider purchasing some (inexpensive) pH test strips to check the alkalinity of their saliva in the morning prior to eating or drinking anything. Ideal results should hover consistently between 7.2 and 7.4.

Using a pulse oximeter is another way to quantify your oxygen uptake. Pulse oximeters can measure your blood oxygen level (O2 saturation) and pulse rate quickly and accurately. Ideally, your oxygen saturation should always be above 95%. Measure your O2 uptake and pulse at regular intervals throughout the day, both during exercise and while at rest.

Staying hydrated. While we seldom stop to think about it, water is made of two hydrogen atoms and one oxygen atom. Drinking an adequate and appropriate amount of water will not only help you stay hydrated, it will increase the amount of oxygen in your blood.

Maintaining an optimal iron level. Normal red blood cells are full of iron, which binds to and transports oxygen from the air we breathe to our tissues and cells. Female athletes (particularly those participating in high-impact sports) have notoriously low iron levels. According to researchers at Harvard University, low serum iron levels (including those that aren't linked to the onset of anemia) are the number one nutritional cause of hypoxemia among women.

Remember to check your iron levels at least once a year to confirm that both your serum iron and ferritin levels are at least in the middle of the 'normal' lab reference ranges. And make it a point to eat plenty of iron-rich foods including beef, liver, lamb, clams, dark leafy greens, and dark (greater than 70%) chocolate.

Slowing down for at least a small portion of the day. While most competitive female athletes will need to engage in higher-intensity training sessions several times a week, research indicates that slow, mindful movement can have a positive impact on cellular health.

Intentional, meditative movements like Qigong, Tai Chi, and leisurely walking all contribute to improved cellular oxygenation.

Remaining active. Try to limit your sitting time to less than three hours a day. If that's not a realistic goal, focus on changing positions frequently. Even the simple act of standing will trigger the beneficial oxygenation of your body. Get up from your chair and do a few quick stretches every 20 minutes and take an active, five-minute break from sitting at least once every hour.

Getting a Massage. Deep tissue massages improve circulation and, therefore, the oxygenation of the tissues and cells. In addition to increasing circulation, massage supports the health of the nervous system and improves lymphatic function, which plays a pivotal role in the mobilization and removal of toxins. In fact, massage enhances every essential physiological process by stimulating fluid and energy movement throughout the body.

Laughing it off. Because laughing sharply increases your oxygen uptake, it can support your cellular health. But improved oxygenation isn't the only benefit. Laughing massages the organs and improves digestion. It strengthens the function of your immune system and facilitates the clearing of accumulated waste products from your cells.

Sleeping in a high-oxygen environment. Consider leaving your bedroom window cracked or open if and when it's possible; a poorly ventilated bedroom can cause hypoxemia. Take steps to address any outstanding issues you may have with obstructive sleep apnea (OSA), which causes dangerously low oxygen levels. In fact, any type of compromised breathing during sleep will compromise your cellular health.

Nitric Oxide: Oxygen's Undercover Partner

Until a few decades ago, researchers paid little attention to the colorless gas molecule known as nitric oxide (NO), and even less attention to its role in human health and performance. Because nitric oxide molecules are so small and have such a short life span (just a few seconds), their critical importance to cellular health wasn't recognized until the early 1990s.

Nitric oxide helps the body's cells communicate more efficiently with one another. NO is essential for optimal health, performance, and recovery because it works as a natural vasodilator—it relaxes and widens the blood vessels which allows blood, nutrients, and oxygen (all the raw materials cells require) to travel through the bloodstream with greater ease. It also supports the immune system, supporting the body's ability to fight off infections. And it serves to facilitate the transmission of messages between nerve cells which contributes to improved memory and learning capacities, better sleep, and a more positive outlook on life.

The amount of nitric oxide found in your body following physical exercise is a reliable predictor of your overall fitness capacity. You can measure and track your nitric oxide level using a simple and relatively inexpensive salivary assessment strip NO test strips can be purchased online at purecleanperformance.com or berkeleywellness.com.

Nitric oxide declines with age.

While nitric oxide levels can be low for a variety of reasons including arterial damage, a lack of dietary nitrates, insufficient stomach acid, imbalanced mouth bacteria, excessive stress (which includes overtraining), the greatest threat to your NO level is your age.

When we're young, our bodies produce large amounts of NO in the endothelial lining of the arteries, which keeps them resilient and pliable. By the age of 40, however, we produce only half the amount of nitric oxide we did at the age of 20. By the time we reach 70, we're capable of producing only 25% of the nitric oxide our bodies need to function fully and efficiently.

 Fortunately, there are a number of things we can do to improve our body's ability to produce NO, regardless of our age.

Begin by using food as medicine; eat plenty of nitrate-rich vegetables. The nitrates that are naturally found in vegetables (especially red beets) are converted into nitric oxide by the body. Since this conversion process begins with the healthy bacteria found in the mouth, make sure you chew your food well and consume any liquids (like soups and vegetable juices) slowly.

The foods with the highest nitrate content are red beets and leafy greens such as kale, arugula, chard, and spinach. Secondary sources include parsley, Chinese cabbage, leeks, celery, radishes, and turnips. One strategy for increasing your intake of nitrates is to add steamed or roasted beets to a protein-based smoothie or other blended beverage.

Using a high-nitrate beet juice powder, however, requires a lot less time and effort. It's also the most reliable and economical way to boost your intake of dietary nitrates. I highly recommend any of the nitrate-certified beet products from PureClean Performance (purecleanperformance.com) which include a 100% organic beet juice powder; a beet-infused performance coffee; a beet-infused chocolate chew; and a powdered, high-nitrate superfood blend that makes a great addition to any smoothie.

Add some polyphenol-rich foods to your daily diet. Polyphenols are a group of beneficial, chemical compounds found in plants. Eating polyphenol-rich foods encourages the endothelial cells found in the arteries to produce more nitric oxide. Red wine, dark chocolate, berries, cherries, pomegranates, chestnuts, and flaxseeds are all high in polyphenols.

Include foods that are rich in vitamins C and E. These vitamins help build and maintain a healthy NO level. The best sources include citrus fruits, broccoli, blueberries, almonds, tomatoes, and green, leafy vegetables.

Optimize your omega-3 to omega-6 ratio. Eat plenty of omega-3 essential fatty acids, found in wild, cold-water fish; grass-fed meats; macadamia nuts, pumpkin, hemp, and chia seeds on a regular basis. Limit your intake of the inflammatory omega-6 fats found in soy, corn, sunflower, safflower, canola, and sesame oils; and the artificial trans fats found in margarines and other processed oils, and packaged foods.

Restore your oral and gastrointestinal health. Healthy bacteria in your mouth and gastrointestinal tract are essential for optimal NO production, so practice good oral hygiene by brushing and flossing regularly. Using plain baking soda instead of a conventional toothpaste will protect and preserve the beneficial, oral bacteria found in the mouth. Strictly avoid the use of any antiseptic mouthwash (which will destroy them) and consider the use of an oral probiotic such as *Bliss K12*.

Add short, high-intensity workouts to your training schedule. They will be more effective than long, slow distance when it comes to increasing nitric oxide in the bloodstream. Exercising at a low to moderate level of intensely for more than 45 minutes will reduce the body's NO supply. In longer, sustained endurance activities, nitric oxide becomes depleted because it's used to support tissue oxygenation.

Rest and recover adequately. And take some time out for yourself each day. Spend as much time as you can outside. Listen to calming music, watch an episode of your favorite TV series, or read a book. If you are spiritual, dedicate a portion of each day to practicing your faith. Just five to 10 minutes of silence a day can improve your body's ability to produce nitric oxide.

Get at least 15 minutes of full-body sun exposure two to three times a week. Many active, health-minded women are aware that getting an appropriate dose of sunlight is critical for optimal health and performance because it fuels the skin's ability to produce an adequate supply of vitamin D3.

While unprotected sun exposure is still actively discouraged by many healthcare professionals, scientific researchers continue to document—in rapidly increasing numbers—its many health benefits. Lower blood pressure, a decreased risk of heart attack and stroke, a heightened sense of wellbeing, improved athletic performance, and a more rapid recovery from both illness and injury are among vitamin D3's many proven benefits. Sunlight plus skin is the body's best source of vitamin D3.

In addition, it turns out that the skin acts as a large storage depot for nitric oxide. Sun exposure plays a critical role in activating the physiological processes that convert the NO that's formed and stored in the skin into the bioavailable form that can be used by the body.

Cellular Requirement #2: Hydration

More than half of what we are made of is water. As an athlete, you already know that it's important to stay adequately hydrated while exercising. But let's take a closer look at the larger role fluid balance plays in the body.

The primary reason we need to drink an adequate amount of water is to keep the blood dilute, which facilitates the quick and easy delivery of nutrients to the hard-working muscles that need them. It also allows for the efficient removal of metabolic waste and heat from them by supporting the body's ability to sweat. More viscous blood not only makes it more difficult for the body to cool itself, it forces the heart work harder. The faster the heart beats, the less effective it is in pumping both blood and oxygen to the tissues and cells.

How much water should you be drinking? It depends. A commonly suggested baseline is 12 cups a day. Since an average of four comes from food, that leaves eight from drinking. Obviously, larger women need more than smaller women. During winter months you'll need less; during the heat of summer and/or if you're exercising, you'll need more.

Your carbohydrate and protein intake will also affect your fluid balance. Have you ever noticed that the word carbohydrate contains the word *hydrate*? For every gram of carbohydrate we store in the form of glycogen, we also store three to four grams of water. So a strict and sudden reduction in carbohydrate calories will result in a corresponding water weight loss. This is how many weight-classed athletes like wrestlers, boxers, and lifters 'make weight.' On lower carbohydrate diets, we naturally store less water. And we store less water when we eat more protein because the body uses it to clear urea (and other waste products) created by protein synthesis.

If you're at all unsure about where your personal hydration status lies on the spectrum of optimal to unhealthy, the simplest thing to do is observe the color of your urine. If it's colorless to slightly yellow, you're hydrated. Gold or dark gold, you need more fluid. Light or dark brown, you're dehydrated.

Keep in mind that about a week before a woman's period starts, her progesterone level increases. This causes her body to hold more fluid in its cells than in its blood supply. Women lose about 8% of their plasma (blood) volume when their progesterone levels are high. So when they're exercising, they have less than the normal amount of fluid they would otherwise have available for urinating and sweating.

The inability to sweat is a significant stressor because it makes temperature regulation more difficult for the body. Women should always add a small amount of (natural) salt to any fluid they're drinking in order to pull water back out of the cells and into the blood, especially during the second half of their menstrual cycle.

Got salt?

All endurance athletes should remain somewhat cognizant of the risk of developing exercise-induced *hyponatremia* (low blood sodium). This is a particularly important issue for women because they are typically lighter and smaller than men.

Hyponatremia is a fluid-electrolyte imbalance that occurs when the concentration of sodium found in the blood falls to an abnormally

low level. In simple terms, that means too much water and not enough salt.

Depending on its severity, the symptoms of hyponatremia can range from bloating, mild nausea, and swollen hands to confusion, seizures, and coma. Although hyponatremia is often associated with prolonged exercise, it can also occur at rest when too much fluid is taken in too quickly.

While excessive drinking is a key risk factor for developing hyponatremia, there are other causes. Ultra-distance athletes, for example, can become hyponatremic from losing large amounts of sodium in their sweat without replacing it.

Aging is also associated with the increased risk of hyponatremia because older women are slower to rid themselves of water when compared to younger women (due to their slower kidney function).

Because of their decreased hormone function, postmenopausal women have particular hydration issues to consider: they don't perform well in the heat because they tend to sweat less and feel less thirsty, which further contributes to their risk of developing hyponatremia.

Good Salt, Bad Salt

While salt has long been demonized as a cause of hypertension, heart disease, and stroke, sodium is an essential nutrient. And like all other essential nutrients, getting enough salt is necessary for achieving and maintaining optimal health. In fact, women who consume an adequate amount of salt tend to enjoy steadier blood sugar levels (because they process insulin better) and greater stress resistance (since salt speeds cortisol clearance from the blood). They enjoy healthier digestion and last—but certainly not least—they tend to live longer.

But not just any salt will do. Refined, white 'table salt' is heated to such an extreme temperature that its chemical composition becomes irreversibly altered. During the refinement process, 82 of the 84 minerals found in natural salt are removed, leaving only two behind—sodium and chloride. Refined salts often contain aluminum, which has been linked to the onset of Alzheimer's disease. Sodium increases blood pressure because it holds excess fluid in the body. Chloride increases the presence of certain forms of thirsty gut bacteria which divert water into the intestines causing diarrhea. The use of table salt will do more harm than good when it comes to supporting and maintaining the body's fluid balance.

Natural and unprocessed salts, however, contain many beneficial minerals. Celtic sea salt and Himalayan crystal salt (harvested 5,000 feet beneath the Himalayan mountains) are both good choices. One difference between sea salts and crystal salts is color. While sea salts tend to be gray, crystal salts are pink.

Nutritional comparisons show that sea salts are lower in sodium and higher in magnesium, phosphorus, and potassium than Himalayan salt. However, Himalayan salt contains considerably more minerals. While crystallized Himalayan salt is considered a more 'pure' form of salt, sea salts are described as 'fresher.'

Real® salt is another, health-enhancing alternative to refined salt that's very similar to Himalayan salt; they both have the full spectrum of minerals and both are considered crystal salts. The biggest difference between the two is geography; Real® salt is sourced from deposits found in the United States near Redmond, Utah. Tasted side by side, Real® salt is slightly sweeter; Himalayan salt has an 'earthier' flavor.

Scientific analysis suggests that Celtic, North, Mediterranean, and Hawaiian sea salts contain fewer microplastics—the tiny particles of petrochemical-based polymers which now contaminate the Earth's lakes, streams, rivers, and oceans.

Dehydration is still a greater concern.

While we've been hearing more about the risk of hyponatremia among women, mild but chronic dehydration (too little water and/or too much sodium in the blood) still merits more attention.

While we can train our bodies to respond to many biological stimuli, we cannot train them to adapt to dehydration. And losing even small amounts of water will affect our energy and athletic performance. In fact, research indicates that just a 1% drop in body water can lead to reduced aerobic endurance.

The good news is that staying properly hydrated doesn't have to be hard. In fact, the most recent research suggests that the safest and most reliable strategy is to forget the calculations and recommendations you may have seen posted on the internet and simply drink when you are thirsty. Of course, it's always wise to remain cognizant of the common symptoms of dehydration which include headaches, dizziness, flushing, and a rapid heart rate.

Is your hydration drink dehydrating you?

Based on the research done by Dr. Stacy Sims, an exercise physiologist who specializes in thermoregulation, hydration, and performance nutrition at the Stanford School of Medicine, it probably is.

"We have this fixation with not bonking, so the industry pumps drinks full of carbohydrates," Sims explains. "But these sugary drinks force your body to move water into the GI tract to facilitate digestion—and out of your blood and muscles."

The end result of the process Sims describes is dehydration. And her suggested approach to fixing it is rooted in simple, common sense. Before the rise of products like *Gatorade®*, athletes separated their hydration from their fueling. Sims encourages athletes to obtain their calories from solid food while satisfying their hydration requirements with liquids.

Plain water will provide well for the body's basic hydration needs. But if you're working hard or going long, you'll need something more (sodium). You'll also need what Sims calls a "driver," a small amount of simple carbohydrate (glucose) that's taken in with sodium. Because sodium can't cross any cellular membranes without glucose, the two work synergistically to provide for an optimal hydration strategy.

Are Sparkling Waters Healthy?

In addition to regulating blood flow, oxygen delivery, and body temperature, water provides us with a source of minerals. Sparkling waters can be a very refreshing source of minerals, but some brands offer more than others. *Apollinaris, Badoit, Borsec, Gerolsteiner*, and *San Pellegrino* are all naturally carbonated mineral waters, each with a unique mineral content and taste. *Gerolsteiner*, for example, is the highest in magnesium; *San Pellegrino*, in beneficial sulfates.

Not all sparkling waters contain naturally occurring minerals or carbonation, however. Many companies infuse their waters with sourced minerals and carbon dioxide. Despite what you may have heard, these beverages have not been proven to be any more (or less) acidic than their naturally carbonated counterparts and they don't leach minerals from the bones.

Some studies show that drinking sparkling water with a meal can increase satiation by encouraging food to stay in the stomach longer. Other studies have shown that it can relieve the symptoms of indigestion and constipation.

One small study of 18 postmenopausal women showed that drinking sodium-rich carbonated water decreased LDL (bad) cholesterol, inflammatory markers, and blood sugar. What's more, they also experienced an increase in HDL (good) cholesterol.

Keep in mind that drinking sparkling water (or any carbonated beverage) might exacerbate the symptoms of irritable bowel syndrome (IBS) and cause uncomfortable bloating. And don't forget to read ingredient labels. Avoid sparkling waters with added sugar or artificial sweeteners (which can acidify the body). Many flavored sparkling waters have hidden ingredients, even if they have no calories.

Cellular Requirement #3: Micronutrients

Micronutrients are the vitamins and minerals our bodies require in small amounts for normal physiological function. While they are needed in much smaller quantities (200 to 1000 times less) than macronutrients, the body needs a wide variety of them—in the correct amounts—to function well.

Since every woman is physiologically unique, each will require different micronutrients in different amounts. Many factors including genetics, age, lifestyle choices, and dietary habits can make a big difference. Women who are still menstruating, for example, will probably need more iron. Those who are under stress will require some additional B vitamins and vitamin C. Women with certain genetic predispositions may need extra folic acid, B12, or glutathione.

What are Vitamins?

Vitamins are organic compounds that play an essential role in growth, repair, digestion, energy production—virtually every metabolic process that happens inside the body. Unlike macronutrients, vitamins don't provide us directly with energy. Since our bodies can't manufacture them, we need to source them from food or supplements. Because vitamins are relatively fragile, they can be inactivated when cooked, stored, and/or exposed to air. As a result, they can have a difficult time making their way into the body.

In general, there are two types of vitamins—fat soluble and water soluble. Fat-soluble vitamins are required to travel through the body bound to dietary fat. Without an adequate supply of healthy fat, the body can't digest, absorb, and utilize the fat-soluble vitamins found in food. Fat-soluble vitamins nourish the body's lipid or fat-based structures including the brain, eyes, and cellular membranes. Because they can be stored in our adipose (fat) tissues, we don't necessarily need to eat them every day. Vitamins A, D, K, and E are all common fat-soluble vitamins.

Water-soluble vitamins can be more freely transported in the (water-based) bloodstream to the body's cells and tissues. Since the body doesn't have a long-term storage mechanism for them, however, they must be eaten regularly. The B vitamins and vitamin C are among the most commonly recognized water-soluble vitamins.

 Food preparation methods will significantly affect how efficiently—or inefficiently—vitamins are absorbed.

This is particularly true when it comes to water-soluble vitamins, which can easily be lost in water during cooking. In general, the best methods for cooking most vegetables are steaming, stir-frying, or roasting. Some vegetables are better absorbed when fully cooked such as those high in lycopene (like tomatoes) and carotenoids (especially carrots). Those high in blue-red compounds (such as red cabbage, plums, and berries) are best absorbed when eaten raw.

Since dietary fat is necessary for absorbing fat-soluble vitamins, consider adding some olive oil or avocado slices to your green salads. While the practice of food combining often requires more time and planning than is practical for many women, be aware that the absorption of some micronutrients can be enhanced or inhibited by the presence of other nutrients found in certain foods. We need vitamin C, for example, to better absorb the iron found in green vegetables. That makes lemon juice and kale a great combination.

What are Minerals?

Minerals come from the earth's surface. Soil and water contain the minerals that plants absorb. Animals eat the plants. Humans eat the animals (along with many plants). **So it should be fairly easy to see why the quality of the soil our food is grown in determines how nourishing it is—or isn't.**

The body uses minerals to perform many different functions—building strong bones, transmitting nerve impulses, carrying oxygen to the muscles, boosting immunity, and supporting cellular health. Some minerals are used to make hormones and oxygenate the cells, others to build bone and muscle, and to maintain a healthy heartbeat.

 Approximately 4% of the body's total mass consists of minerals, and they all need to be sourced from food, water, and/or supplements.

Since minerals are already in their simplest form (they are elements), the body doesn't need to break them down in order to absorb and utilize them. And minerals aren't damaged by oxygen or heat. Since they can survive any method of cooking, they are readily available to the body. They do, however, need to bind to other things—like amino acids—so that they can be used effectively.

Some foods contain minerals bound to oxalic acid (like leafy greens, nuts, black tea, and chocolate) or phytic acid (found in beans, whole grains, nuts, and seeds) which make them harder to absorb. But that doesn't necessarily mean these foods should be avoided.

Those who have a predisposition for developing kidney stones, however, should avoid oxalates.

Since phytates can bind and inhibit the absorption of minerals, women who have iron-deficiency anemia or difficulty building or maintaining their iron stores should make it a point to limit their intake of beans and grains.

Minerals: The Macro and the Micro

Minerals are classified into macrominerals (those we need more of) and microminerals (those we need less of).

Macrominerals are present at larger levels in the body and are required in larger amounts in the diet. They include calcium, chloride, magnesium, phosphorus, potassium, sodium, and sulfur. Daily requirements and recommendations can be as high as 1,000mg of magnesium for women who are deficient.

Macrominerals provide the body with the basic materials it needs to make its electrochemical processes (like nerve impulses) happen. As a result, these materials are commonly known as electrolytes. Athletes need an adequate supply of electrolytes for contracting and relaxing muscles, balancing body fluids, and maintaining healthy nerve cell function.

Microminerals are often referred to as "trace minerals" since they are required in very small amounts. They include chromium, cobalt, copper, fluorine, iodine, iron, manganese, molybdenum, selenium, and zinc. Daily requirements of these are as little as 200ug for selenium and chromium (5,000 times less than magnesium) and as high as 25mg for zinc.

Minerals should be balanced.

Maintaining a proper mineral balance is essential for optimal physical and mental health. If your calcium level is a lot higher than your magnesium level, for example, you'll be more prone to muscle cramps. Zinc and copper imbalances have been increasingly inked to attention and mood disorders.

Keep in mind that certain foods can inhibit the absorption of certain minerals. For instance, the tannins and polyphenols found in coffee and tea can inhibit iron absorption. Foods (or beverages) high in vitamin C, however, can promote it.

While all minerals are important for optimum health and performance, the two major minerals—calcium and magnesium—are the true 'overachievers.' In addition to building and maintaining strong bones and teeth, calcium supports healthy heart, muscle, and brain function. Magnesium regulates enzymatic activity (which drives every chemical reaction happening inside the body), energy production, and cellular reproduction. It's important to note that magnesium and calcium must act jointly in controlling many physiological processes. Healthy muscular function, for example, requires both calcium (which causes tension in the muscle fibers) and magnesium (which relaxes them).

Magnesium: The King of Minerals

The importance of magnesium for athletes has been thoroughly studied and the results are very clear: it's necessary for optimal health and performance, regardless of what kind of athlete you are. Magnesium supports optimal neurological, cardiovascular, and muscular strength, efficiency, and recovery. It also works synergistically with vitamin D3 to reduce inflammation, build strong bones, and strengthen the immune system. As an added bonus, it prevents unwanted calcification in the joints.

Athletes have a higher baseline need for magnesium because it's excreted through sweat and used for both energy production and muscular recovery—requirements that naturally increase with higher levels of physical activity. Studies suggest that strenuous exercise increases the body's need for magnesium by at least 20%.

Do you remember learning about how light energy from the sun fuels the process of photosynthesis in your high school biology class? As it turns out, this process is magnesium dependent. Magnesium enables plants to convert light into energy. Since animals and humans obtain their food supply by eating plants, the entire food chain begins with magnesium. Chlorophyll, the 'life blood' of plants, is virtually identical to the hemoglobin found in our red blood cells. The only difference is that chlorophyll contains a magnesium atom which makes it green and hemoglobin, an iron atom which makes it red.

After oxygen, food, and water, magnesium is the most critical element present in the human body. A full three-fourths of all enzyme production is magnesium dependent, including the production of adenosine tri-phosphate or ATP—the basic energy currency of the body.

Other processes controlled by intracellular magnesium include:

- The contraction and relaxation of all muscles, including the heart and blood vessels
- The transmission of messages along nerve cells
- The creation, repair, and protection of DNA and RNA
- The regulation of cellular metabolism
- The stabilization of blood sugar and insulin
- The production, absorption, and utilization of vitamin D3

Unfortunately, the average American gets only about 40% of his or her recommended daily allowance (RDA) of magnesium. Remember: the RDA is the absolute minimum standard for preventing disease, not for optimizing health and performance.

In addition, the American diet is high in protein and calcium, which both increase magnesium excretion and the body's need for even more of this essential mineral. High amounts of phosphorus (common in processed meats, sodas, and energy drinks) bind dietary magnesium, making it difficult to absorb. Add to this the excessive use of caffeine, sugar, table salt, and alcohol; mental and physical stress; chronic pain, low thyroid function, high blood sugar, and heavy sweating and it should come as no surprise that 90% of the U.S. population is suffering from an unrecognized magnesium deficiency.

From an evolutionary perspective, the human body became adapted to a diet that included a plentiful supply of magnesium. So it didn't need to develop a strong or efficient mechanism for processing or storing it. As a result, magnesium is both poorly absorbed and easily excreted.

Obviously, female athletes are at a greater risk for becoming magnesium deficient than their sedentary counterparts. A marginal magnesium intake coupled with an increased magnesium demand (created by strenuous exercise, injuries, mental and emotional stress, and the sweat-induced loss of magnesium) can lead to a severe deficiency. In fact, a severe magnesium deficiency is one of the often-unrecognized reasons why seemingly healthy, young athletes die suddenly from heart arrhythmias.

The bottom line? It's absolutely essential to eat magnesium-rich foods on a regular and ongoing basis. Best sources include:

- Green leafy vegetables (chard, spinach, and kale)
- Raw cacao and dark chocolate (greater than 70%)
- Nuts and seeds
- Vegetables (peas, broccoli, cabbage, green beans, asparagus, and Brussels sprouts)
- Seafood (salmon, mackerel, and tuna)
- Legumes (black beans, chickpeas, and kidney beans)
- Fruit (fresh figs, avocados, bananas, and raspberries)

In addition to eating more magnesium-rich foods, almost all female athletes will benefit from taking 250mg of supplemental magnesium daily. I can recommend Jigsaw Health *MagSRT,* Life Extension *Extended Magnesium,* and Ancient Minerals *Magnesium Oil Spray.* In addition, consider taking a 20-minute soak once or twice a week in a hot bath with two cups of Epsom salt (magnesium sulfate). Epsom salt baths are not only a great way to relax, but an excellent source of transdermal (through the skin) magnesium support.

Calcium: The Queen of Minerals

If magnesium is the king of minerals, calcium is the queen—especially for women since they run a much higher risk of developing osteoporosis than men. As a general rule, women have a lower bone density than their male peers and lose bone mass more quickly as they age. Although there are other possible genetic and environmental factors that can contribute to bone loss, the female body's changing level of estrogen is the usual suspect.

Estrogen is a hormone that helps regulate a woman's reproductive cycle. At the same time, it plays a role in keeping bones strong and healthy. While premenopausal women have more estrogen than men, they will experience a dramatic drop in estrogen production during menopause. They are more likely to experience bone loss and osteoporosis at that time.

But menopause isn't the only cause of estrogen-related osteoporosis. The risk is increased among women who experience irregular or infrequent periods, or began having their periods at a later than normal age. Women who have had their ovaries removed (at any age) are also more likely to suffer from osteoporosis.

 Calcium is an important bone-building mineral, but calcium supplements aren't a quick fix for osteoporosis.

In fact, they can often do more harm than good. In her book, *Better Bones, Better Body*, Dr. Susan Brown writes, "Over and over we are told to consume adequate calcium. What we are not told, however, is that we also need other bone building nutrients."

If you regularly follow health and fitness news, you may have heard about the studies linking the use of calcium supplements to higher heart attack rates. Despite what you may have been told, taking calcium without its companion nutrients—magnesium, vitamin D3, essential fatty acids, silica, and vitamin K2—can be harmful.

The problem with calcium is that it doesn't travel straight from our glass of milk or serving of yogurt into our bones, despite what the American Dairy Association would like us to believe.

Without its companion nutrients, calcium won't be properly absorbed or utilized by the bones or any other living tissue. If there isn't enough vitamin D3 to drive the absorption process correctly, for example, all the calcium intended for the bones and teeth will end up being taken in by (and hardening) the arteries.

Unfortunately, heart disease isn't the only health problem that can be attributed to excessive calcium. Increasing your calcium—without simultaneously increasing your magnesium—can lead to the formation of calcium deposits in the joints (leading to arthritis) or kidneys (leading to kidney stones).

It's important to note that the countries with the highest calcium intake (over 1,000 milligrams daily) have the highest osteoporosis rates. In fact, populations that consume only a few hundred milligrams of supplemental calcium (but obtain an abundant supply of other key nutrients from their diets) suffer from little to absolutely no osteoporosis and have the lowest bone fracture rates.

Why? High calcium intake interferes with the absorption or utilization of many nutrients including manganese, magnesium, iron, zinc and phosphorus—minerals that bones need to become strong and remain flexible.

The Milk Myth

The 'milk myth' is based on a belief that this calcium-rich drink is required for healthy bones. But as memorable and likable as the "*Got Milk?*" campaign has been, it's time to stop listening to what the dairy industry has been telling us all these years.

Milk does contain a fair amount of calcium, but so do almonds, dark leafy greens, and fish. Several scientific studies have actually shown a number of detrimental effects linked to milk consumption. The most surprising of these is poor calcium absorption. As it turns out, we don't absorb the calcium found in cow's milk all that well, especially after it's been pasteurized. In fact, milk consumption has been shown to drive calcium out of the bones.

Pasteurized milk acidifies the body which, in turn, triggers a biological correction. Calcium is an excellent acid neutralizer and the biggest storage of calcium in the body is found in the bones. So the very same calcium that our bones need to stay strong is pulled from them in order to neutralize milk's acidifying effects.

That's not to say there isn't room in a healthy diet for milk products, especially those that are fermented, like yogurt and cheese. **And it's important to keep in mind that not all milk is created equal.** Raw, full-fat milk from grass-fed animals can be a nutrient-dense, whole food for those who can tolerate it. Think of pasteurized and/or homogenized milk as more of a processed food.

As Chris Kresser, an internationally recognized leader in ancestral health, paleo nutrition, and functional medicine, explains, "In a sign of nature's wisdom, raw milk contains lactase, the enzyme needed to digest lactose. Pasteurization, however, kills lactase. So if you don't produce your own lactase, you'll have a hard time digesting pasteurized milk."

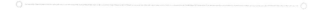

 As is the case time and time again when it comes to defining what foods are 'good' or 'bad' for our health, performance, and recovery, there are no hard and fast rules.

There are many women who are lactose-intolerant or otherwise sensitive to milk protein, which means that they have trouble digesting it and aren't necessarily absorbing the calcium it contains. If pasteurized milk products aren't consumed along with an adequate supply of alkaline-balancing foods, their acid-forming actions can promote calcium loss. While dairy products do contain a great deal of calcium, they're a small part of a much bigger picture. For optimal bone health, consider implementing at least a few of the following suggestions:

- **Rebalance your calcium intake.** If you're concerned about maintaining healthy bones, skip the supplements and focus on getting an adequate and balanced amount of calcium from your diet.

    There are many calcium-rich vegetables that do 'double duty,' supporting bone health while alkalinizing the body. These include the cruciferous vegetables—broccoli, cauliflower, Brussels sprouts, green and red cabbage, collard and mustard greens, kale, bok choy, Swiss chard, watercress, turnips, rutabaga, and radishes.

    If you don't have any digestive issues with dairy, its moderate intake can help with building and maintaining healthy bones. But remember that salmon contains more calcium, vitamin D3, and vitamin K2 than milk. So even if you've got milk, get some salmon, too. Other excellent sources of calcium include almonds, broccoli rabe, butternut squash, chia seeds, clams, kelp, leafy greens, and sardines.

- **Let the sun shine in.** Our bodies were meant to be exposed to a health-enhancing amount of sun. For most women, 15-20 minutes of full body sun exposure during peak daylight hours two to three times a week will allow the body to make an adequate supply of vitamin D3, which encourages calcium absorption. Try to allow yourself a few hours before showering with soap after a sunbath; it will strip the newly manufactured vitamin D3 from the surface of your skin before it can be absorbed.

If you don't live in a climate that allows for year-round sun exposure, supplement with some additional vitamin D3. Research has consistently shown that 1,000–5,000iu per day is a safe and adequate dose. Because the process of digestion interferes with vitamin D3 absorption, sublingual sprays and/or drops are typically more effective.

Make sure to assess your vitamin D3 level regularly (ideally with every change of season) to make sure you're not over or under supplementing. At-home test kits are widely available online (at purecleanperformance.com) and in some pharmacies.

- **Increase your intake of vitamin K.** Add more green, leafy vegetables and fermented foods to your daily diet. And consider the use of a vitamin K2 supplement, unless you're taking a blood-thinning medication like *Coumadin®*. I can recommend Life Extension's *Super K*.

- **Monitor your estrogen level.** Estrogen plays a big role in the maintenance of bone mineral density and overall bone health. Bones get weaker and lose density during menopause. A woman's risk of osteoporosis, fractures, and other bone-related incidents skyrocket during and after her transition. Then, maintaining an adequate intake of bone-building nutrients becomes even more critical.

- **Strength train,** especially as you get older. In fact, regular strength training should be considered an essential activity for any woman over the age of 45. Most women reach their peak muscle mass sometime during their late 30s or early 40s. After that point, a gradual loss begins. While sedentary women can lose 3-5% of their total muscle mass each decade after the age of 30, those who stay active preserve more. Stronger muscles mean stronger bones—and a healthier metabolism.

- **Incorporate some rhythmic motion** into your training or recovery regimen. Recent research has confirmed that our bones are living tissue that can thrive and grow at any age—as long as they are stimulated by weight-bearing force and rhythmic motion. While running can get the job done, it's actually not as effective as rebounding (lightly jumping up and down on a standard or mini trampoline).

When done correctly, rebounding places just enough pressure on bones to stimulate the production of new cells and the absorption of calcium. Just 10-15 minutes of rebounding three times a week can be highly effective in preventing (and even reversing) bone loss. Since it can be done without the risk of adding weight-bearing stress to the knees, ankles, hips, and back, it's even something that non-runners or injured athletes can do to strengthen their bones and muscles.

- **Assess the status of your bone health.** Bone resorption testing is becoming more widely used as an accurate and inexpensive way to measure the rate of bone loss when compared to a DXA or dual-energy x-ray absorptiometry bone density scan.

Many functionally oriented physicians are now also using laboratory assessments such as the *urine NTX* or the *serum CTX* tests as valuable tools in the early evaluation and prevention of osteoporosis. These tests offer an opportunity for practitioners to identify rapid or excessive bone loss before too much damage has occurred. They also allow for the more regular and frequent assessment of a woman's bone health status than bone density scans can practically provide.

Iron: Another (Really) Important Mineral

Iron deficiency is one of the most commonly identified nutritional disorders. And it's particularly prevalent among female athletes.

Iron is an essential health and performance nutrient because it's required to produce *heme*, a key component of the hemoglobin found in red blood cells. Hemoglobin is what binds and carries oxygen from the lungs to the muscles. If your hemoglobin level is low, your muscles won't receive as much oxygen and your health and performance will suffer. In addition, iron is fundamental to the proper function of many other physical systems. It's necessary for good bone and tissue health, for example; and it serves as a catalyst for the production of aerobic energy.

Low iron levels are a world-wide health concern that's becoming increasingly common among children and teens, those who follow a vegan or vegetarian diet, and menstruating women. Endurance athletes (especially runners) are also prime candidates for iron deficiency. The causes of low iron are many, the most obvious of which include:

- **A low dietary iron intake.** The typical endurance athlete eats more grains, fewer fats and meats (which are a great source of highly absorbable heme iron), and fewer *non-heme* (the form of iron available in fruits and vegetables) foods like spinach, beet greens, and bok choy.

- **Iron loss on foot strike.** The force of the foot hitting the ground initiates the breakdown of red blood cells. High-mileage runners and those who run or play their sports on hard, paved court surfaces are especially at risk.

- **Iron loss through sweat and urination.** Although a relatively small amount of iron is lost through sweat and urine, athletes who regularly train and/or compete in hot, humid conditions or have a propensity to sweat more profusely than others are at an increased risk.

- **Iron loss through the gastrointestinal tract.** The loss of iron through small, normal, and otherwise inconsequential bleeds into the stomach or large intestine is actually quite common. While they don't represent a health risk, they do contribute to a cumulative iron loss.

Symptoms of iron deficiency include:

- Poor performance and slow recovery
- Exercise fatigue and/or lethargy
- Increased heart rate
- Heavy or stale legs
- Susceptibility to infection
- Irritability
- Ice cravings
- Reduced mental acuity and memory

Phytonutrients and Myconutrients

In addition to vitamins and minerals, the body needs the phytonutrients found in plants and the myconutrients found in edible fungi (including lichen and mushrooms). These compounds not only act as powerful antioxidants, they support healthy hormonal function. If you use a natural progesterone cream, its source is likely the wild yam. In addition to repairing our DNA, phyto and myconutrients fight off bacterial and viral infections, improve intercellular communication, reduce chronic inflammation, support detoxification—and so much more.

Some of the more well-known phytonutrients include:

Carotenoids, which are a large group of several hundred, fat-soluble pigments widely found in plants and animals. Their intake has been linked to a decreased risk of certain cancers, stroke, heart disease, and eye disorders. Carotenoids are also thought to enhance the immune system. The carotenoids that have been most studied in this particular application are beta-carotene, lycopene, lutein, zeaxanthin, and astaxanthin.

Chlorophyll is a green pigment found in almost all plants and algae. This powerful phytonutrient can regenerate our bodies at the cellular level and has been shown to help fight infection and heal wounds. It may also support the body's circulatory, digestive, immune, and detoxification systems. Chlorophyll consumption increases red blood cell production and, therefore, heightens the body's ability to use oxygen.

Flavonoids, also called "bioflavonoids," are a group of naturally occurring compounds found in vegetables, berries, fruits, and cacao.

They exhibit strong antioxidant and anti-inflammatory properties. And they add both color and flavor to fruits and vegetables.

Catechins or flavanols are found in onions, apples, berries, red wine, broccoli, tea, coffee, and cocoa beans. Clinical studies have shown that the consumption of certain flavanol-rich foods such as chocolate, green tea, and red wine can result in improved cardiovascular function.

Some of the most well-studied myconutrients include:

Chanterelle mushrooms, which have high concentrations of B vitamins, play a role in helping the body convert food into energy and in keeping the nervous system functioning well. Chanterelles are high in fiber, which supports regular bowel function and good gut health. They have antimicrobial, antibacterial, and antifungal properties and are rich in both vitamin D3 and potassium.

Chaga mushrooms contain large amounts of an antioxidant-rich pigment known as melanin. Various studies have shown that chaga can help control or prevent diabetes, cardiovascular disease, immune dysfunction, and DNA damage. This particular micronutrient has been consumed for centuries in the East, usually as tea, where its health benefits are well-established

Maitake mushrooms are an important ingredient in traditional Chinese and Japanese medicine, used for health and longevity. They have been researched extensively and found to contain several anticancer, antiviral, and immune-enhancing agents. They have also been used to treat high cholesterol, manage both high and low blood pressure, and improve blood sugar stability.

Button mushrooms, the world's most commonly eaten myconutrient, have grown wild and been eaten by humans since the days of the early hunter-gatherers. Modern-day studies have shown button mushrooms to be effective in preventing breast cancer.

Many ancient civilizations knew that mushrooms contained special properties. The ancient Egyptians believed mushrooms could grant immortality, so only the pharaohs were deemed worthy of eating (or even touching) them.

Cellular Requirement #4: Antioxidant Protection

The majority of phytonutrients are also antioxidants. Since large amounts of antioxidants are naturally found in plants, eating a wide range of fresh produce should become (or remain) a top priority.

The origin of all plant life is the sea. When species of marine plants began adapting to life on land, they also began to produce non-marine antioxidants such as ascorbic acid (vitamin C), polyphenols (beneficial plant chemicals) and tocopherols (vitamin E). They did this in an effort to protect themselves from their newly developed need to utilize the oxygen in the air (a process known as oxidation).

This defense mechanism is what originally caused plants to become pigmented. Pigmentation acts as a beneficial biological defense against the free radical damage that's caused by photosynthesis (the energy production process used by plants). When you eat more color, you are consuming more antioxidants.

When eaten in combination, micronutrients and phytonutrients not only provide cellular nutrition but have the synergistic ability to act as antioxidants, protecting your cells from the harmful effects of free radical damage or oxidation (the unavoidable consequence of any metabolic process). Just as metal rusts and a slice of apple browns in the presence of oxygen, free radical damage triggers changes in the structure of otherwise healthy cells.

It's quite common to see charts that take a reductionist approach to classifying foods based on their antioxidant content. For example:

Vitamin A. Dark green vegetables such as broccoli, spinach, turnip greens, carrots, squash, sweet potatoes, pumpkin, cantaloupe, apricots, liver, eggs, and dairy products.

Vitamin C. Citrus fruits and their juices, guava, kiwifruit, papaya, berries (especially strawberries), mangoes, pineapple, red peppers, parsley, broccoli, cauliflower, watercress, tomatoes, and liver.

Vitamin E. Nuts, seeds, non-glutinous whole grains, green leafy vegetables, kiwifruit, olive oil, avocados, and fish oils.

 Unfortunately, this isolated approach can reinforce a too narrow view of the way antioxidants really work. Antioxidant protection is a team effort.

In order to be protected, we need to consume the tens of thousands of plant-based antioxidants that our bodies have evolved to use. The only real way to pump up your antioxidant protection is by increasing the variety of colorful (preferably organic) produce you eat.

Even if you've got the 'healthy diet' thing down, it can still be tough to provide for all of your body's nutrient needs. Many fruits and vegetables (including organics) are picked before they are fully ripe, which reduces their total nutrient content. Commercial farming practices have depleted the trace minerals found in soil—and in our food. Our busy, on-the-go lifestyle means that we don't always take the time to eat well-balanced, nutrient-dense meals. While we might get a few (maybe even quite a few) of the 'macros' and 'micros' we need, it's probably not happening 100% of the time. So there can be a place for a multi-vitamin supplement made from fresh, whole-food concentrates.

Because the human body is designed to thrive on foods, not chemicals, it doesn't recognize or absorb synthetic and/or isolated supplements well. In recent years, several large-scale studies have actually been called off when researchers determined that certain synthetic supplements had the opposite effect of their naturally occurring counterparts found in food.

 While research supporting the use of dietary supplements is mixed, volumes of scientific studies have confirmed the health and performance benefits of eating whole, nutrient-dense foods.

Oxford University, for example, completed a long and rigorous study of 20,000 subjects in the UK. The study reported no substantial beneficial effects from the use of high-potency vitamins C, E, and beta carotene. But a whole-food diet was strongly correlated with positive, long-term health outcomes.

The Journal of Diabetes Care published a study concluding that vitamin E supplementation had no effects on slowing the progress of chronic disease; foods that were rich in vitamin E did. The *Journal of the National Cancer Institute* reported similar findings in the study of plant-based carotenoids; they had no benefit when they were isolated and used alone, but quite beneficial when eaten in whole-food form (as carrots).

The list of studies goes on and on, but the overwhelming conclusion from all of them is pretty much the same—supplementing with synthetic and/or isolated micronutrients isn't helpful and might even be harmful. Because micronutrients are engineered to work together, taking a lot of one can disrupt the balance of all the others.

In the interest of allowing the body to achieve a solid and sustainable micronutrient balance, avoid the use of any synthetic combinations or isolated forms of vitamins and minerals (which eliminates 99.9% of the big-name grocery store and pharmacy brands). If and when you have an identified nutrient deficiency, choose a product made from whole-food concentrates. While an isolated vitamin C supplement contains one active ingredient (ascorbic acid), an orange contains this along with 172 other supportive compounds. It doesn't exactly require advanced math to figure out that you'll receive more antioxidant benefits from eating an orange than taking a synthetic ascorbic acid supplement.

Why are antioxidants so important? The creation of free radicals is a natural process that happens continuously throughout the body, and a steady supply of antioxidants are required to neutralize their harmful and unavoidable effects.

While the body is capable of producing some of its own antioxidants, supporting your cells with targeted foods or supplements made from whole-food concentrates during periods of increased physical and emotional stress can be beneficial. Maintaining a high antioxidant level becomes even more critical as we get older since the body's ability to make its own antioxidants declines with age.

Zoonutrients: What Animals Offer

The final category of micronutrients that should be recognized are the *zoonutrients*—the micronutrients found in animals. The most important players include conjugated linoleic acid, CoQ10, and creatine in red meat; colostrum, alpha-lactalbumin, and lactoferrin in dairy proteins; growth factors, certain essential sugars, and cholesterol in lightly cooked egg yolks; type II collagen in chicken cartilage, and nicotinamide adenine dinucleotide or NAD+ in fermented dairy products. A healthy and balanced intake of zoonutrients can reduce the risk of heart disease, support healthy brain function, and speed muscular repair. In general, the most nutrient-rich sources of zoonutrients will come from animals raised under the best circumstances: organic, pasture-raised beef and chicken, and wild-caught fish.

Collagen is an especially important zoonutrient. While collagen won't directly prevent or speed the healing of an injury to an athlete's tendons and ligaments, it can be a very beneficial supplement when viewed from an amino acid standpoint. Glycine is the primary amino acid found in collagen.

Glycine supports the body's ability to break down and utilize nutrients like glycogen (stored glucose) and fat to create energy. In the process, it also supports the muscular, immune, digestive, and nervous systems. Since the body can manufacture a certain amount of glycine, it's considered a non-essential amino acid. However, it can only make about three grams a day—not nearly enough to satisfy the body's minimum requirements (which is about 10 grams), let alone the extra demand created during any kind of injury or recovery process.

 Our primitive ancestors enjoyed eating entire animals for breakfast, lunch, and dinner, including their glycine-rich ligaments and tendons. Since we no longer do that, we're missing out on the supply of glycine that was once so abundant in our daily diets.

Some additional benefits of collagen supplementation include increased levels of glutathione, the amino acid that protects against oxidative damage. Research shows that it can also improve sleep quality by decreasing core body temperature and increasing cutaneous blood flow. Especially for women, a cooler body temperature encourages deeper sleep. Studies show that three grams of glycine taken before bed can improve sleep quality and reduce the daytime drowsiness that occurs after a poor night of sleep.

There are a variety of ways to add glycine to your diet. Bone broth (now available in many grocery stores) contains approximately 27 grams of glycine per 100 grams of protein. It also contains several other amino acids and additional nutrients which act synergistically to enhance their combined absorption.

These key nutrients include:

- **Chondroitin and glucosamine**, which have been shown to support the integrity, elasticity, and mechanical properties of cartilage.
- **Hyaluronic acid**, which is the main component of synovial (joint) fluid.

- **Proline**, which forms the structure of collagen and, like glycine, is another conditionally essential amino acid. Athletes recovering from injuries have a higher need for proline.

Mixing up a batch of fruit-juice-sweetened gelatin blocks or making some gelatin-based desserts (use yummly.com as a recipe resource) are two additional strategies for adding more glycine to your diet. Get creative in the kitchen: collagen and gelatin can also be easily added to smoothies, soups, sauces, homemade ice cream, and baked goods.

 Since it wouldn't be enjoyable to create meals with the sole objective of maximizing their micronutrient content, focus on eating the widest possible variety of unprocessed plant and animal foods. Make it your mission to eat a rainbow of color every day.

How to Make Your Own Bone Broth

Bone broth is a satisfying and delicious medicinal food that's quite easy (and very economical) to make at home. While the making bone broth does take time (about three hours in an Instant Pot® or up to two days using more traditional methods), it requires very little preparation time or effort. **For the highest collagen content in your broth, start with bones that are full of connective tissue.** Use necks, feet, backs, joints, and knuckles whenever possible. The carcass from a whole, roasted chicken or remnants of a roast or spare ribs will also make an excellent bone broth.

If you don't have any left-over bones at home, meat vendors at farmer's markets or butcher shops will often sell their remnant bones inexpensively. Always opt for the highest quality bones you can find—organic, free-range, grass-fed, and local.

The key to getting the best flavor from the bones you use is to make sure they are cooked or roasted first. If you are using bones from leftovers you can skip this step, but raw bones should be roasted at 425°F for 25-30 minutes, or until very brown.

Cover the bones and scraps generously with filtered water and let the whole mixture soak for about 30 minutes prior to cooking. Adding two tablespoons of apple cider vinegar to the mix will help break down the bones more quickly. After cooking for three hours in an Instant Pot® or 24 to 48 hours using a slow cooker or stovetop, you'll have bone broth.

Make sure you simmer the broth at a very low temperature if you're working with a stovetop. Use the smallest burner at the lowest setting after first bringing it to a boiling point over medium heat. If you don't feel comfortable letting the broth cook on a burner overnight, it's fine to take it off, let it cool, and store it in the refrigerator overnight. Re-start the simmering process again in the morning. Poultry bones should simmer for 24 hours; bones from red meat for 48 hours.

Once cooked and cooled, you can strain the bone broth through a fine, mesh sieve (or colander lined with cheesecloth) and either enjoy or pour into glass jars for storage in the refrigerator or freezer. A layer of fat will solidify at the top of the broth after chilling You can discard it or scoop it off and use it like any other cooking oil. Or, you can simply mix it back into the reheated broth. If you freeze your broth, make sure you don't fill your jars all the way to the top (it will expand when frozen). The broth should also become gelatinous when cooled. The thicker the broth, the more collagen it contains.

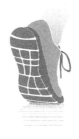

Obstacle Four

Digestive Dysfunction

While we spend a lot of time and place a great deal of emphasis on figuring out how much of which foods we should (or shouldn't) eat, it's what we absorb from the food we eat that ultimately matters most. Unfortunately, women suffer disproportionately from a number of conditions that interfere with their ability to assimilate the nutrients found in food.

 Women experience more digestive dysfunction than men. In fact, they are twice as likely to suffer from a gastrointestinal disorder than their male counterparts.

We know that women produce less stomach acid than men, which means they digest their food more slowly and less efficiently. Studies done by the Mayo Clinic confirm the marked difference in digestion time between men and women. Based on their research, it takes about 47 hours for food to travel through the large intestine of women compared to 33 for men. This may be due to the fact that women have a longer colon, by an average of almost four inches. This anatomical difference may be attributed to the female body's need for more water to create amniotic fluids during pregnancy.

We also know that the ovaries and the uterus are located below the intestines in a woman's anatomy. Since they are such close neighbors, conditions affecting the female reproductive organs may also affect the intestines. Endometriosis, for example, is a collection of uterine tissue that grows outside the uterus, sometimes causing an intestinal blockage. Women who suffer from endometriosis often report symptoms of diarrhea, constipation, or bloating—especially during their periods.

Hormonal imbalances can also contribute to digestive difficulties.

In many ways, the female hormones (estrogen and progesterone) work in conjunction with the digestive system to keep it working smoothly. If their levels become deficient or imbalanced, digestion is often affected. Both estrogen and progesterone can influence the movement of food through the intestines—sometimes speeding the process up, causing diarrhea, nausea and abdominal pain; at other times slowing it down, causing gas, bloating, and constipation.

Perimenopausal women are particularly prone to digestive dysfunction. As a woman's body prepares for menopause, the production of her estrogen and progesterone levels fluctuate and eventually decline. Low female hormone levels have been conclusively linked to the onset of IBS (irritable bowel syndrome) and a number of other digestive difficulties including poor motility (intestinal movement) and increased visceral hypersensitivity (intestinal pain).

DIGESTIVE DYSFUNCTION

Women who are under a great deal of stress can also suffer from a wide range of digestive difficulties due to the larger amounts of cortisol circulating through their bloodstream. Increased cortisol levels interfere with digestion by raising both blood pressure (which directs blood away from the stomach where it's needed for digestion) and blood sugar (which can result in dizziness, headaches, increased thirst, and nausea); by slowing down the release of stomach acid; and by delaying the movement of digested food into the small intestine.

In addition, cortisol modulates the regions of the brain that stimulate cravings for high-sugar and/or high-fat foods, both of which quiet the stress response by triggering the release of soothing serotonin when eaten.

First Things First

In order to put all of the potential energy and nutrients found in food to work, the body first has to digest it. And digestion is complicated, for men and women alike.

Because our food was once another complex, living thing (either plant or animal) it's chemically complicated and has to be simplified through the process of digestion. The word digestion comes from the Latin *digerere*, which means to separate or divide. And that's exactly what our digestive system does—it breaks food down into its macro and micronutrient components, then separates and sends them where they're needed.

Digestive disorders are incredibly common. While that doesn't make them normal, some are relatively easy to solve. Bloating, belching, nausea, dyspepsia, and passing undigested food particles in the stool, for example, are often caused by eating too fast. Chewing prompts the brain to send signals to the entire digestive system, preparing it for action. If you don't chew your food properly, you won't digest your food properly. It's as simple as that.

Making sound food choices is another relatively uncomplicated solution to many common digestive complaints. Packaged foods, refined sugars, and alcoholic beverages frequently cause problems and are devoid of any real nutritional value. Because they consume so many nutrient resources for their own processing, they end up leaving few—if any—behind.

Problems like heartburn and acid reflux are often blamed on excess stomach acid, but they are typically caused by pressure from the backup of poorly digested food and resulting overgrowth of bacteria. Ironically, the problem isn't too much stomach acid, it's too little. And using an antacid to suppress the symptoms will only make matters worse.

Some distance running coaches actually advocate the use of an antacid prior to longer or more difficult workouts to help ease and prevent exercise-induced nausea (caused by a buildup of acid as blood flow is directed away from the stomach lining and to the legs). There are a number of reasons not to do this. In addition to promoting bacterial overgrowth and excessive gas, the use of antacids impairs nutrient absorption, protein digestion, and immune function.

A number of other digestive difficulties are found further down the digestive chain.

The small intestine is where most of what we eat is converted into its usable forms—glucose (from carbohydrates), amino acids (from proteins), and fatty acids (from fats). It's also where the body decides if it can recognize and use certain food particles or if it should classify them as an antigen—a bacteria, virus, toxin, or other pathogen. Food allergies are created when inadequately digested food proteins are mistakenly identified antigens. The most common offending foods are sometimes those eaten with the greatest frequency and/or those that are difficult to digest.

If you suffer from recurring bouts of diarrhea after eating a meal, a food allergy may be causing your digestive system to reject its contents too quickly; your body is attempting to flush out what it perceives as a harmful irritant—along with all the other contents of your small and large intestines.

Celiac disease is an increasingly common digestive disorder caused by a severe intolerance to gluten. When the body mistakenly identifies gluten as an antigen, it wages an all-out war inside the small intestine. The destruction includes damage to the villi—the finger-like projections in the small intestine responsible for absorbing the nutrients found in food. When the villi are damaged, the body can't absorb the raw materials it needs for energy, growth, maintenance, and repair.

According to the most recent statistics, women account for 60-70% of all celiac disease diagnoses. But many researchers believe that at least a third of the total population is unknowingly gluten intolerant. Even in the absence of an (identified or unidentified) intolerance, there are a number of reasons why avoiding gluten (and grains in general) can lead to improved health, performance, and recovery.

The Case Against Grains and Beans

 All grains and beans contain anti-nutrients—dietary compounds that interfere with the digestion, absorption, and utilization of other nutrients. The four primary anti-nutrients found in grains and beans are gluten, lectins, phytates, and saponins.

Gluten is a type of protein that's most commonly found in all varieties of wheat, rye, and barley. It's also a common allergen, but even those who aren't allergic can still have an intolerance—an inflammatory response to eating it. In addition to causing digestive difficulties and irregular bowel function, a gluten intolerance can surface in myriad ways from bumps on the back of arms, dizziness, hormonal imbalances, and migraines, to mood swings, chronic fatigue, fibromyalgia, and joint pain.

Wheat has the highest gluten content of any grain. And modern wheat varieties differ in several ways from those eaten by early humans. In fact, they have been hybridized and modified hundreds of times over to make them grow faster with less water and become more pest resistant. The wheat sold in the U.S. today is a dwarf variety and distant relative of what our primitive ancestors ate that's significantly higher in gliadin—an appetite stimulant. And it contains an opioid polypeptide that binds directly to receptor sites in the brain, mimicking some of the effects of pharmacological opiates. This is one reason why some women can literally become 'addicted' to eating wheat-based breads, pastas, cereals, and snacks. Modern wheat varieties also cause *agglutination*—the clumping of red blood cells—which greatly increases an athlete's risk for developing blood clots.

While wheat contains the most gluten, all grains contain some type of undesirable protein. Oats, for example, contain avenin; corn contains zein, and rice, orzenin.

Lectins are phytochemical toxins that plants make as a natural defense to radiation, insects, disease, and being eaten. While some plants are programmed to reproduce by having their seeds eaten, fertilized, and redeposited by animals, others propagate by being blown by the wind. Acting as mild toxins, lectins discourage animals from eating these windborne plants (which include both grains and beans).

An animal that consumes lectins is subject to their harmful effects, although tolerance can be built over a long period of time. Since humans have only been consuming grains for about 10,000 years (which represents a tiny fraction of our evolutionary timeline), the lectins they contain still have a toxic effect. Our bodies have simply not had enough time to adapt to them.

Phytates are indigestible compounds found in grains, beans, nuts, and seeds that bind easily to important and necessary minerals like iron, zinc, magnesium, and calcium. Phytates offer some health benefits (they contain antioxidants) when eaten in small amounts, but can deplete nutrients when consumed in excess. Vitamin A, C, and B12 deficiencies, for example, are common in underdeveloped populations that rely heavily on grains and beans as a primary source of calories. Cooking, soaking, sprouting, or fermenting can reduce the phytate content of grains and beans considerably.

Nuts also contain phytic acid. But since we eat them in much smaller quantities than grains and beans, they are less concerning—especially when eaten in the context of a nutrient-rich diet that contains ample amounts of animal-based minerals and protein, which counterbalance the harmful effects of the phytic acid (phytates) found in plants.

Keep in mind that the complete elimination of all phytates from the diet isn't recommended, even if it were possible. There are some health benefits associated with a minimal to moderate phytic acid intake. Research studies show that phytic acid can inhibit calcium crystallization and prevent kidney stones; bind to iron and serve as natural treatment for hemochromatosis (the tendency to absorb too much iron). They might even prevent some forms of cancer.

Beans (or legumes) contain anti-nutrients called *saponins*, which are aptly named because they foam like soap when shaken with water. While saponins provide plants with a natural, chemical defense against microbes and fungi, they can compromise human health. According to Robb Wolf, author of *The Paleo Solution*, "Saponins are so irritating to the immune system that they are used in vaccine research to help the body mount a powerful immune response."

In general, beans contain fewer anti-nutrients and are more nutritious than grains. But they are a less-than-optimal food source, especially for the health-and-performance-minded female athlete.

 Both grains and beans contribute to the onset of leaky gut syndrome.

The cumulative and combined impact of eating large amounts of grains and beans often leads to the debilitating damage of the lining of the intestinal tract and the onset of intestinal hyperpermeability or *leaky gut syndrome*.

Essentially, small perforations in the lining of the small intestine allow undigested food particles, toxic waste products, and bacteria to leak through the intestines and into the bloodstream where they travel freely throughout the body. In an effort to fight back, the immune system attacks them as if they were pathogens. This immune response can result in a wide range of symptoms including digestive difficulties, chronic fatigue, joint pain, muscle aches, poor endurance, chronic inflammation, and delayed recovery from an illness or injury. While mainstream medicine doesn't recognize leaky gut as a diagnosable condition, volumes of scientific evidence support its validity.

Intestinal Flora Imbalances

Thanks to recent research, we now understand that the gut is a highly evolved microbiome (collection of micro-organisms) that serves as the body's 'second brain.' That means the specific types and ratios of organisms found in your intestines determines how your body utilizes food—whether it's used for immediate energy or stored for future use; recognized as a source of beneficial nutrients or rejected as a pathogen. A woman's gut microbes can even cause food cravings by influencing her taste receptors. Researchers have determined that the intestines of women who crave chocolate, for example, contain different bacteria colonies than those who don't—and that food cravings can be eliminated when a particular bacteria population isn't fed.

 The dramatic increase in gastrointestinal disorders has been conclusively linked to the over prescription of antibiotics, which kill both disease-causing bad bacteria and health-enhancing good bacteria.

Like it or not, the inside and outside of our bodies are populated by all kinds of bacteria, both beneficial and harmful. In fact, the bacteria in our bodies outnumber the cells in our bodies by about 10 to one. Most of these bacteria live in the gut.

In a healthy digestive system, the beneficial bacteria render the harmful bacteria benign. And they are always on duty, manufacturing vitamins and persistently patching the intestinal lining in order to prevent pathogens from entering the bloodstream. This restorative activity accounts for about 80% of the immune system's total workload. Ironically, antibiotics reduce the efficacy of the immune system by eliminating good gut bacteria—the body's front-line disease defense. The use of a probiotic supplement should always be considered after the use of an oral antibiotic.

The use of probiotics has become increasingly popular

And for good reason. These beneficial intestinal bacteria work by controlling and balancing the populations of microorganisms living in the intestines. They drive down the numbers of harmful bacteria, improving digestion, immunity, central nervous system activity, and hormone health.

In Greek, the word *probiotic* translates into 'for life.' In addition to the many physiological benefits they deliver, probiotics appear to have an equally positive influence on our psychological health. Research studies have shown them to be effective in reducing the incidence and severity of:

- Depression
- Anxiety
- Fatigue
- Poor stress tolerance

- Mood swings
- Bipolar disorder

Setting all other benefits aside, supporting and encouraging the growth of good gut bacteria may be the key to better digestion. In general, whole foods—not supplements—are always the preferred form of probiotic support. They are more easily absorbed and, as a result, more effectively utilized.

It's important to eat a variety of live cultures from an assortment of fermented foods like kombucha, yogurt, sauerkraut, cheese, pickles, apple cider vinegar, and kimchi.

The Problem with Probiotics

The probiotic puzzle can be difficult to piece together since no two women house the same strains, amounts, or ratios of intestinal flora. But new scientific evidence suggests that certain strains of 'friendly' bacteria offer universal benefits.

Two of the major issues with many popular probiotics are their temperature sensitivity and their inability to survive the body's harsh, digestive environment.

Bacillus probiotics, however, are hardy, spore-based bacteria that are heat stable and capable of surviving the harsh, acidic passage through the stomach and into the gut. While Bacillus strains have been used in probiotic formulations in Europe for over 50 years, they have only become available in the U.S. during the last decade.

Spore-based probiotics come from the soil, which humans have been interacting with since time began. We evolved eating food covered with it, and getting our hands and bodies dirty with it. So it should not come as a huge surprise that our immune systems have learned how to benefit from it.

Bacillus microbes are an integral part of our natural intestinal flora, so our bodies are very adept at using them. In fact, their absence can disrupt normal immunity and metabolism. *MegaSporeBiotic*™ is a particularly good spore-based probiotic that doesn't require refrigeration and even works to restore and re-balance intestinal flora during a course of antibiotic treatment.

In an effort to protect the probiotic populations living in your gut, it's best to avoid antibiotics, anti-inflammatory medications, refined sugars, artificial sweeteners, and processed foods. All of these increase the prevalence of *Firmicutes*—the intestinal bacteria or microbes that are most efficient at extracting sugar from carbohydrates. When this bacterial population becomes dominant, it becomes easier for the cells to derive energy from otherwise indigestible starches, which promotes fat storage.

What's the difference between prebiotics and probiotics? Prebiotics are non-digestible forms of carbohydrates that feed probiotics, allowing them to flourish. In addition to supporting the general health of the gut biome, the use of prebiotics may increase calcium absorption and bone mineral density, particularly in postmenopausal women. Cooked and cooled heirloom potatoes, Jerusalem artichokes, garlic, onions, leeks, asparagus, oatmeal, apples, plantains, and slightly under-ripe bananas are all good prebiotic sources.

The Rise of Irritable Bowel Syndrome

The incidence of IBS is on the rise among women. And recent research has linked its onset to insufficient and/or imbalanced intestinal flora. More specifically, it appears that decreased levels of the beneficial bacteria strains Lactobacilli and Bifidobacteria and increased levels of harmful E. coli and Clostridia have been found in the fecal samples of an overwhelming majority of IBS patients. There are several factors that may lead to microbiome imbalances which pave the way for the onset of IBS. These include the use of antibiotics, a past or current infection, improper dietary choices, and stress—both mental and physical.

Research has revealed that many IBS patients experience a heightened and/or prolonged stress response. They also demonstrate what's known as *visceral hypersensitivity*; they are very aware of the physical sensations they are experiencing at any given moment. This predisposes them to paying even more attention to their IBS-related symptoms, increasing their general level of anxiety and creating a vicious circle.

Research into both Celiac Disease and IBS have brought significant attention to the fundamental importance of healthy gastrointestinal function and the essential role it plays in human health and wellbeing. The recent and rapid rise in the scientific study of gut health may very well make it the next new medical frontier.

Unidentified Food Sensitivities

Food sensitivities are an often-overlooked stressor that reduces the body's overall health and performance potential. Their effects begin with increased inflammation, which can contribute to the onset of any illness or injury. They are also notorious for interfering with healthy digestion and impeding the absorption of nutrients.

According to Theron Randolph, the father of environmental medicine, an overwhelming majority of adults suffer from some kind of food sensitivity. And nine out of 10 of them don't realize that their symptoms are related to the food they eat on a regular (if not daily) basis.

While we typically think about food sensitivities in the traditional sense (sneezing, hives, sinus congestion, and difficulty breathing), they can also surface as anxiety, depression, joint pain, asthma, acne, bad breath, constipation, diarrhea, fatigue, hyperactivity, dark circles under the eyes, and stubborn weight loss.

But food sensitivities differ from food intolerances and allergies.

A food *allergy* exists when the body has an immediate adverse reaction to a food. These reactions can be minor (sneezing) or major (swelling that closes the airway). Many people have very minor reactions to eating foods they are allergic to, which makes them difficult to diagnose.

A food *intolerance* exists when the body lacks specific enzymes to digest a particular food. Gluten and dairy are the two most common food intolerances. Both can cause significant gastrointestinal distress because the body can't properly process them.

A food *sensitivity* is often grouped with a food intolerance, but this condition exists when your body has an adverse reaction to a food anywhere from 45 minutes to three days after you've eaten it. It's estimated that up to 80% of all adults have some kind of food sensitivity and they appear to be more common among women than men. The vast majority of them remain unidentified because the cause and effect relationship between a food that's eaten and a symptom that develops is extremely difficult to establish given that the time lag between the two can be several hours to several days.

 Food allergies, intolerances, and sensitivities often remain unrecognized because their symptoms are normalized.

Having an intermittent but continuously runny nose, recurring headaches, or frequent elimination urgencies isn't normal, but some women accept these symptoms as ordinary or unremarkable.

How do you know if you have a food allergy, intolerance, or sensitivity?

The gold standard for identifying any of these food-related issues is an elimination diet which requires the systematic removal and re-introduction of foods, making note of any positive or negative changes in symptoms (such as joint pain, headaches, skin rashes, nasal congestion, digestive difficulties, or poor sleep). Most elimination diets involve a 21 or 30-day elimination period followed by the gradual and progressive re-introduction of foods. There are also three-day rotational diets, which are more convenient and easier to implement but less exacting and accurate. The *Whole30®* is currently one of the most popular elimination diet programs.

If you're not quite ready to commit to an elimination diet but think you might have some food sensitivities, consider using an app like the *Bulletproof® Food Detective* or measuring your HRV (Heart Rate Variability) prior to and again at one hour after eating a suspect food. If your HRV declines significantly during this time, it means that your sympathetic nervous system has been activated; something you ate is having an adverse effect on your body.

You can also use the following checklist to jump start your informal assessment process:

1. **Do you often think or say, "I couldn't live without pasta, bread, cheese, or___?"** Feeling dependent on any food is a red flag. While your first exposure to a food allergen may be unpleasant as your body struggles to reject it, the stress of the allergic response promotes a release of the body's natural opiates. Repeated exposures to an offending food can lead to adaptation. Even after the allergic symptoms subside, the release and effects of the feel-good opiates continue—and become addictive.
2. **Despite eating a well-balanced diet and getting plenty of exercise, do you have a difficult time staying lean?** When you're eating foods that don't work for your body, you inevitably develop chronic inflammation which promotes fat storage.
3. **Do you struggle with water weight gain?** Do your hands, fingers, feet, and ankles tend to swell? These are often signs of food-related inflammation. When you're inflamed, you'll retain water and be more prone to swelling.
4. **Despite being fit, do you wish you were in better health?** Regardless of your best efforts, do you have to manage a variety of nagging issues that range from gas and bloating to low energy, delayed recovery, constipation, anxiety, insomnia, and headaches?

5. **Does your 'seasonal hay fever' seem to last all year long?** A runny nose, dry eyes, and sinus congestion are all signs of seasonal allergies, but if you suffer from these symptoms most of the year, you could be dealing with a hidden food sensitivity.

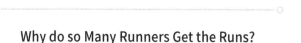

Why do so Many Runners Get the Runs?

Doctors and researchers don't know exactly how many female runners suffer from exercise-induced diarrhea, but they estimate that it afflicts a third to a half of those who are training or competing at any given time.

One reason for the distress could be that the digestive organs aren't getting enough blood during exercise, a condition known as ischemia. In the body's ongoing attempt to maximize its resources, the heart pumps oxygen and nutrients to the organs and systems that need them the most. During a long or intense run, the skin and large muscles are the most deserving recipients; the intestines become a lower priority. In this instance, our glutes have more of a need for oxygenated blood than our stomachs. In fact, during a peak physical effort, blood flow to the internal organs can decrease by as much as 80%. The resulting lack of blood flow to the intestines can make them more prone to malfunction.

The frequent use of non-steroidal anti-inflammatory drugs (NSAIDs) such as ibuprofen may also be triggering or exacerbating the problem. While there is a place for their occasional use (for pain and inflammation), they can cause problems anywhere along the GI tract, from the esophagus to the colon. In a healthy gut, the epithelial cells in the gastrointestinal tract hold tightly together, preventing undigested food particles and other pathogens from entering the bloodstream. NSAIDs make the mucus lining the intestines more permeable, increasing the risk of gastritis (intestinal inflammation) and ulcers (small sores on the stomach lining). Since non-steroidal anti-inflammatory drugs work partly through reducing blood flow to the digestive system, their harmful effects should be considered carefully by athletes. One study found that damage markers in the digestive system were twice as high in runners who took anti-inflammatory medications compared to those who didn't.

It's likely that dietary choices, however, play the most important role in the incidence of digestive distress many otherwise-healthy female athletes experience during or after exercise. A large and growing body of evidence against the reliance on 'healthy whole grains' is compelling. And it's not just because they are high in dietary fiber (a common and well-recognized cause of diarrhea). Nature designed the outer husks of all grains to be protective, arming them with a mild toxin known as phytic acid. Unlike berries and other plants that rely on being eaten in order to reproduce, grains were designed to propagate by being blown by the wind. In order to survive, they need to avoid being eaten. This explains why their protective defense mechanism (the shell or husk) is toxic.

The best and simplest way to know if grains (or beans) are causing you any digestive distress is to completely eliminate them from your diet for at least 21 days. If this fails to provide relief, you may be suffering from an undetected food sensitivity; from leaky gut syndrome, or intestinal inflammation.

Gut Health, Inflammation, and Immunity

 Chronic inflammation has been linked to the onset of digestive dysfunction—and almost every other known illness.

As a result, it's starting to receive some serious attention within the realm of conventional medical research. Since conventional medicine focuses on treating symptoms instead of addressing the root cause of an illness or recurring injury, this research represents a promising new horizon in both the treatment and prevention of disease. Arthritis is an inflammation of the joints. Heart disease is an inflammation of the arteries. It appears that the conventional medical community is beginning to realize that figuring out how to reduce chronic inflammation in the body may be a better solution than using medications to reduce joint pain or lower cholesterol.

It's important to remember that inflammation isn't always bad; it's essentially the body's pre-programmed course of protection. There are, however, two distinctly different types of inflammation—acute and chronic. Acute inflammation is a localized response (typically to an injury) characterized by increased heat and a collection of fluid that initiates a healing response. Unless severe trauma is involved, it starts quickly and generally disappears in a few days.

Chronic inflammation, on the other hand, can last for weeks, months, or even years if its cause isn't identified and eliminated. This type of inflammation isn't the result of immediate trauma; it's a slow and insidious process that keeps the body locked in a state of constant repair. Immune cells (macrophages, monocytes, and lymphocytes) are always at work, alternately destroying and rebuilding tissues in an effort to rid the body of its inflammatory offenders.

Neutrophils (white blood cells) also become involved in the inflammatory response, attacking what they perceive as outside invaders by producing and spreading a large dose of free radicals throughout the body. And they will continue with this defensive process for as long as they detect any inflammation. Their erratic and assaulting behavior can lead to the destruction of healthy cell walls and, eventually, damaged DNA. The body's general immune response is also reduced when it's taxed by and preoccupied with fending off the incessant, harmful effects of inflammation—especially in the intestinal tract.

The intestines are an important part of the immune system because they prevent foreign substances from entering the body. In fact, gastrointestinal tissue accounts for almost 80% of all human immune tissue. When chronic inflammation compromises GI function, the entire immune system suffers.

At this point, it should be fairly clear to see that the human immune system isn't an external barrier that somehow surrounds and protects the body. Rather, it's a complex internal hub of defensive activity centered in the digestive system. **Sound intestinal health is the foundation of a strong and resilient immune system.**

Digestive Health and the Brain

Both 'gut feelings' and 'butterflies in the stomach' are sensations that offer some fairly conclusive evidence that the brain and digestive system are biochemically connected. This connection is known as the *gut-brain axis*. Recent studies show that the health of each system is dependent on how well the two can communicate together.

Their conversation begins with neurons, the cells found in the brain and central nervous system that tell your body how to behave. There are 100 billion neurons in the human brain and another 500 million found in the gut (the body's *second brain*). The vast network of neurons found in the intestinal lining form the enteric nervous system which is directly connected to the brain by the vagus nerve. The vagus nerve is a cranial nerve that connects the brain to the body.

The gut is not the site of higher-level cognition (like solving mathematical equations or even reading this book); it exists more in the realm of intuition and instinct. Scientific research has now established that the *enteric* (pertaining to the gut) nervous system responds to emotions by sending a variety of brain chemicals known as neurotransmitters to the brain via the vagus nerve.

When the adrenal glands release cortisol (the fight or flight hormone), for example, the gut responds by releasing serotonin (the happy hormone) in an attempt to protect both brain and body from the harmful effects of stress. Ninety-five percent of the body's supply of serotonin is actually manufactured in the gut. Based on this information, we know that the health of a woman's enteric (intestinal) nervous system plays a key role in determining how well she can cope with physical and mental stress.

Gamma-aminobutyric acid or GABA is another calming neurotransmitter produced by the tiny but intelligent microbes living in the intestinal tract. Studies in laboratory mice have shown that the use of certain pre and probiotics can increase the production of GABA, which reduces anxiety, depression, and mood swings.

The gut microbiome collectively creates a number of other beneficial chemical compounds. Some are neurochemicals that heighten mental clarity, learning, and memory. Others are short-chain fatty acids like propionate, which has been linked to improved cardiovascular health; acetate, which promotes increased fat metabolism; and butyrate, which quells intestinal inflammation.

The restorative actions of butyrate also bolster the immune system's ability to contain the spread of systemic inflammation by curtailing the distribution of pathogens throughout the body. When inflamed, the gut becomes leaky, allowing undigested food particles, bacteria, toxins, and other undesirable materials to enter the bloodstream where they feed the inflammatory process. By healing the intestinal tract and stopping the leaks, butyrate helps the immune system function more optimally.

 Since intestinal flora communicate directly with the brain, improved gut health may lead to improved psychological health.

Certain probiotic strains are known to have a direct, positive impact on mental health. In addition to supporting the gut-based synthesis of neurotransmitters (such as serotonin, GABA, and dopamine), these *psychobiotics* can reduce stress hormones (especially cortisol), suppress brain inflammation (by keeping cytokine levels in check), promote the growth of new brain cells (by increasing levels of brain-derived neurotrophic factor or BDNF), and protect the brain from free radical damage (by acting as antioxidants).

Certain prebiotics have also been shown to positively affect brain health, so be sure to include higher-fiber fruits and vegetables (like artichokes, asparagus, bananas, beets, broccoli, jicama, and leeks) in your diet. **In addition to supplementing with pre and probiotics, there are some relatively simple things you can do to help your gut-brain axis communicate more effectively. These include:**

1. **Supplementing your diet with omega-3 fatty acids.** These healthy fats are found in oily fish like mackerel and salmon. Studies in both humans and animals show that omega-3s can support the growth of beneficial gut bacteria, which reduce the risk of certain brain disorders.
2. **Eating more fermented foods like yogurt, kefir, sauerkraut, and raw-milk cheese.** In addition to improving digestive health, fermented foods can fight food allergies, improve cognitive function, and boost immunity.
3. **Including a wide variety of polyphenol-rich foods in your daily diet.** Cocoa, green tea, olive oil, and coffee all contain polyphenols—plant chemicals that encourage the growth of healthy gut bacteria.
4. **Eating more tryptophan-rich foods.** Tryptophan is an amino acid that is converted to serotonin—the calming neurochemical made in the gut. High-tryptophan foods include turkey, eggs, and cheese.

Digestion: Why the Mind Matters

The digestive process doesn't begin in the mouth; it begins in the brain the moment we become consciously aware of our hunger. And it remains in charge of the entire digestive process once we begin to eat. The brain manages every stage of digestion, alerting each organ system (from the mouth to the colon) to prepare for incoming food and nutrients. This sequential, step-by-step process is more specifically managed by the autonomic nervous system (ANS) and it's two branches—the sympathetic (fight or flight) system, and the parasympathetic (rest and digest) system.

The gastrointestinal or GI tract responds to signals from both branches of the ANS. With intense activity or stress, the sympathetic nervous system (SNS) shuts down both digestion and appetite. If you think about the hours and minutes leading up to a competitive event, you probably don't feel hungry; your mouth may go dry and you might even feel 'butterflies' in your stomach. That's the SNS at work.

The parasympathetic nervous system (PNS) promotes the calm and consistent action of digestion. In situations of extreme fear or trauma, however, the SNS response can become exhausted, causing the PNS to suddenly activate. Since intestinal motility is one of its primary, digestive functions, a spike in parasympathetic activity can cause the loss of bowel or bladder control.

It's quite clear that the nervous system plays a decisive role in the digestive process. And this has an impact on determining what many athletes can (or can't) eat before an event or difficult training session. It also influences what food choices an athlete makes following a competition or difficult workout.

When to eat can sometimes be a more important consideration than what to eat.

If you've just completed a tough training session, it's best to wait at least 30 minutes before eating solid food in order to extract the most nutrients and obtain the most restorative benefits from it. If you're working with a recovery window of less than 30 minutes, it's better to opt for a liquid form of nutrition since the digestive system will still be working under sympathetic control. On moderate to difficult training days, consider postponing the intake of any food for at least 30 minutes following a workout. Your body will benefit more fully from food when your digestive system has settled back into its parasympathetic mode.

Think about it. Whether your body is in an acute, sympathetic mode from being physically challenged or from an increased level of mental or emotional stress, make a conscious effort to activate your parasympathetic system when you eat. Try to avoid eating while you're standing or moving, browsing the internet, or driving your car. Your thoughts, feelings, and environment all affect nutrient processing.

Becoming aware of how you're feeling and what you're thinking while you're eating is an important, first step in maximizing your body's ability to fully extract and assimilate the nutrients found in food.

Are You a Hypochondriac?

Long before medical practitioners had a clear understanding of the mechanisms that cause disease, it was believed that most physical ailments started in the stomach. The ancient Greeks called this *hypochondriasis*.

Breaking the word *hypochondria* down into its Latin roots, we have *hypo*, which means below, and *chondria*, which refers broadly to cartilage and more specifically to the ribs. When the two roots are combined, we are left with a word that literally means 'below the ribs.' This area of the body is, of course, the gut.

With the advent of the microscope, scientists began to see and understand things like bacteria, parasites, and viruses—information which allowed doctors to link the onset of an illness to a more tangible and definitive cause. In time, the meaning of the word hypochondria as a medical term changed. In more recent years, the word *hypochondriac* has been used to describe a person who has a persistent and often-inexplicable fear of having a serious medical illness.

As it turns out, the ancient belief that illness begins in the gut may ultimately prove to be more accurate. We now know that many chronic illnesses are either caused or exacerbated by gastrointestinal dysfunction.

Gut Health and Autoimmune Disease

The incidence of autoimmune disease is increasing at an alarming rate. According to the National Institute of Health, 23.5 million Americans suffer from some form of autoimmune disease (although some believe that number is actually closer to 50 million). There are nearly 100 different, diagnosable autoimmune diseases recognized worldwide—with more being identified every day. And their primary target is moving beyond those above the age of 50. Young women in their 20s and 30s are now frequently being diagnosed with autoimmune conditions such as lupus, rheumatoid arthritis, type 2 diabetes, Hashimoto's thyroiditis, psoriasis, and inflammatory bowel disease.

 The rise of autoimmune-related diseases can be attributed to poor dietary choices, chronic stress, and a leaky gut.

Medical experts have also established a link between the increased incidence of autoimmune disease and the more frequent use of C-section deliveries.

Babies born vaginally swallow a big dose of their mother's microbiome as they pass through the birth canal. Those delivered by

C-section miss out on being inoculated with all the beneficial bacteria found there. Instead, their first exposure tends to be to the bad bacteria found on the skin or in the mouth of the adults who hold and kiss them. The most recent research shows that C-section babies are more likely to suffer from food allergies and an imbalanced gut microbiome.

Studies have also shown that even before birth, a mother's use of antibiotics can permanently impact her baby's gut biome. And infants naturally inherit their mother's microbiome—healthy or not. But nature, in her infinite wisdom, provided women with the ability to nurse their young. Breast milk contains a wide variety of naturally occurring probiotics and anti-inflammatory compounds which can override the bad bacteria and encourage the good bacteria to flourish.

By adulthood, 80% of the human immune system has been firmly established in the gut. So it's important to protect and nurture it by making sound and supportive food choices. The Standard American Diet or SAD (which is high in processed grains, sugars, and unhealthy oils and low in fiber, vegetables, and antioxidants) has been conclusively linked to poor gastrointestinal health.

 Remember: inflammation begins in the gut and autoimmune disease begins with inflammation.

Eliminating SAD foods will be an important first step in eliminating bad (inflammatory) gut bacteria and reducing intestinal inflammation. Identifying (and avoiding) foods that trigger an allergy or sensitivity can be helpful, too. Support the growth of good gut bacteria by eating plenty of pre and probiotics.

Another great way to support gut health is to incorporate bone broth into your diet. The amino acids lysine and glycine along with the collagen found in bone broth all help repair the gut lining, which will improve the immune system over time.

No Guts, No Glory?

Recent research has shown that gut bacteria influence how well an athlete performs and how quickly she recovers. In fact, it appears that the presence of certain intestinal microbes may provide a competitive edge.

> Intestinal microbes are not only responsible for how efficiently we break down macronutrients, absorb micronutrients, and create energy, they regulate stress resilience, neurological function, and willpower—key variables influencing optimal athletic performance.

Even the specific type of sport an athlete tends to excel at has been linked to the presence or absence of particular gut microbes. In a 2019 study conducted by Harvard University, researchers sampled the gut microbiomes of athletes training for the Boston Marathon. Following the event, they found a spike in a certain strain of bacteria among the group's top performers. The scientists believe that populations of this particular bacteria (Veillonella) increased because its preferred food source is lactic acid. Distance runners who have large amounts of Veillonella living in their intestinal tract may be more successful because they experience less lactic acid build up.

In another study, Harvard researchers compared the gut microbiomes of rowers and ultra-marathoners. The significant differences they found in each group's microbiome composition suggests that the pursuit of certain sports may foster the development of specific microbial ecosystems. These findings have prompted researchers to search for ways to manage the microbiome for enhanced sports performance and recovery. The pivotal role microbes play in energy regulation and athletic aptitude have researchers exploring questions like:

- Could microbiome mapping and editing help us predict (or create) the next great athlete?
- Could (or should) we harvest the microbes of elite athletes in order to pass on (market) their performance-enhancing microbial capabilities?
- Is it ethical to alter an athlete's existing gut microbiome through the use of performance-enhancing probiotics, or would this practice provide an unfair advantage?

Exercise and the Microbiome

Although food is the most influential factor determining the breadth and depth of microbes living inside the intestinal tract, exercise can play an important and positive role—as long as it's not excessive. An excessive amount of physical exercise can cause dysbiosis (an imbalance of the body's microbiome), an underlying cause of both injury and illness.

Thanks to recent research, it has become infinitely clear that the composition of intestinal microbiome populations exist on a spectrum, with sedentary microbes at one end and very active microbes at the other. **The key is to determine the amount (and intensity) of physical exercise that's right for your body and your microbiome.** The answer often requires a great deal of personal experimentation. **When optimized, however, there are nine different ways a healthy and balanced microbiome can positively impact athletic performance:**

1. **Reduced Inflammation.** The gut microbiome plays a significant role in inflammation, either increasing or decreasing its level. While acute Inflammation serves a productive and protective purpose, chronic inflammation interferes with athletic performance; it slows recovery and is the root cause of most chronic illness While dysbiosis is associated with inflammatory conditions, research shows that a balanced microbiome can reduce systemic inflammation, providing both short-term symptom relief and long-term disease risk reduction.
2. **Improved Energy.** When your gut microbiome is balanced and diverse, it becomes easier for your body to create energy. When your body is more efficient at producing energy, you'll look, feel, and perform better.
3. **A More Positive Attitude.** Because the microbes found in the gut are capable of 'talking' to the brain through the vagus nerve, they play a significant role in determining your state of mind. Dysbiosis has been linked to both mood disorders and mental illnesses, especially anxiety and depression. On the flip side, a healthy gut microbiome can contribute to a more positive—and focused—mind. The gut-brain axis influences mental fortitude, which is an essential prerequisite for optimal athletic performance.
4. **Better Body Composition.** A healthy and diverse microbiome will improve the body's ability to run smoothly and efficiently. When the gut microbiome is in balance, it makes staying fit, lean, and healthy more effortless. This is largely because it positively influences the body's metabolism and composition (ratio of muscle to fat).

5. **Stronger Bones.** The microbiome helps build bone mass and strength through hormone and immune system regulation. A balanced gut microbiome can improve the bone-mineral absorption of calcium and magnesium. A properly balanced microbiome can also speed the healing of broken bones.
6. **Improved Nutrient Absorption and Utilization.** When a woman's gut microbiome works well, her entire body benefits. A balanced microbiome is especially important when it comes to the digestion, absorption, and utilization of food. If the gut microbiome is imbalanced or unhealthy, then its microbes will spend the majority of their time simply fighting to survive; they won't have the time or energy to process nutrients properly.
7. **Healthier Hydration.** A diverse and balanced microbiome has been linked to more consistent hydration levels, and the more efficient use of water during exercise. A healthy microbiome also helps to maintain the integrity of the intestinal lining, which is a key variable influencing proper hydration.
8. **Improved Sleep.** Dysbiosis is associated with poor sleep and impaired cognition. This is because the gut microbiome controls the production and distribution of hormones such as cortisol, serotonin, and GABA which all affect sleep quality. The microbiome also influences the production of melatonin, which is essential for proper sleep-wake cycles.
9. **Stronger Antioxidant Activity.** You have an impressive, albeit invisible, antioxidant defense system stored inside your body. Athletes depend on this system to keep them performing and recovering consistently well. A healthy and balanced gut microbiome will support and strengthen the body's antioxidant defenses. In fact, their combined cooperation can help prevent exercise-induced tissue damage; it can lower oxidative stress, reduce both physical and mental fatigue, and improve athletic performance.

Exercise can improve the microbiome making it easier to stay strong, lean, and fit. But like many things in life, too much of a good thing can be a bad thing. Avoid overtraining for optimal intestinal health.

What can you do to improve the health of your intestinal microbiome?

Take steps to expand its diversity. A diverse microbiome means a healthy microbiome. Eating a wide variety of foods is essential. But you can take this strategy to the next level when you eat foods that have been specifically selected to satisfy your body's unique microbial needs. This is exactly what a *Viome*® assessment does. *Viome*® uses an RNA-sequencing technology along with artificial intelligence to develop a list of personalized food recommendations that will optimize the breadth and depth of your intestinal microbiome.

A *Viome*® assessment requires the collection of a small fecal sample which is sent to the lab using a pre-paid envelope. The cost has become increasingly affordable over the past few years. An assessment should be performed at least twice a year for best results. A doctor's prescription is not required.

Examining Excrement

This section should be considered optional for anyone who might have a difficult time pondering poop. Taking a closer look at what you're depositing in the toilet, however, can provide you with a lot of information about your digestive system. While most people assume that their solid waste is the used-up remains of digested food, it's primarily water and intestinal bacteria—most of which is still alive. It also contains fiber and other indigestible plant matter (like cellulose) and small amounts of tissue including old cells from the intestinal lining that have been sloughed off during digestion.

 The specific texture, shape, and color of your stools can point to things like dehydration, undetected illnesses, and dietary deficiencies.

If your stools are black or tarry (and you haven't been using supplements that contain iron, charcoal, black licorice, or bismuth), white, or they contain blood, see a doctor to rule out the possibility of a more serious illness. Ideally, your feces should be colored brown by stercobilin (a normal by-product of red blood cell breakdown) and bile (which helps digest fat). When stercobilin is not present, poop takes on a pale grey or whitish color (a symptom of liver disease or clogged bile ducts).

Picture-perfect poop is medium brown in color, solidly formed in the shape of a snake, and passed both easily and regularly once or twice a day. If the color varies or you can see pieces of food that you recently ate, you may be eating too quickly, have low stomach acid, or a food intolerance.

When runny or generally unformed, variable in color, and showing foods you've recently eaten in a clearly identifiable form, your body may be trying to rid itself of an infection or you've eaten something it's reacting to and wants to get rid of—fast. If the reaction is strong enough that it causes you to suffer from a bout of diarrhea (multiple instances of a loose stool over the course of a day or several days), it will be important to repopulate your gut with pre and probiotics. Under normal circumstances, it can take anywhere from one to three days for food to be completely digested and its waste products eliminated.

If your poop is dark and formed into small balls or pellets, you are likely experiencing an intestinal flora imbalance, dehydration, or stress. It could also be that you're not eating an adequate amount of soluble fiber. Drinking more water and adding a few more probiotic foods and root vegetables to your daily diet should improve your overall digestive health.

When shaped (but thicker and more difficult to pass) and medium to dark brown in color, take note of how many processed proteins—powders, bars, or even meats—you've been eating. Consider trading at least some of them in for real food such as wild-caught fish, pasture-raised eggs, or grass-fed steak.

If your poop is yellow, green, or very light in color and/or tends to stick to the sides of the bowl, you've probably eaten more processed (or even healthy) fats than your body can digest. If this is a persistent problem, you may want to consider having your gallbladder checked as it may not be releasing an adequate amount of (fat-digesting) bile. A yellow stool can indicate the presence of giardia, a microscopic parasite.

If it's dark in color with a strong odor and sinks to the bottom of the bowl, the likely culprit is too many processed foods. It could also suggest that your body is struggling to clear itself of external toxins—from personal care products, plastic packaging, bottled water, food storage containers, household cleaners, and the environment. Make an effort to limit your exposure to plastics and chemicals; and drink plenty of water. You'll find more information in an upcoming chapter on how to identify and eliminate hidden toxins.

Completing a stool analysis (like *GI Effects* from Genova Diagnostics or *GI-360* from Doctor's Data) is the best way to gain the most accurate and comprehensive insights.

A stool analysis can help pinpoint any digestive dysfunction, intestinal inflammation, and/or microbiome imbalances that may be compromising your gastrointestinal health. These panels offer a multifaceted assessment of many chronic, digestive concerns. Frequent and ongoing bouts of diarrhea, for example, could be caused by a variety of different problems including digestive enzyme insufficiency, intestinal inflammation, food allergies, or the presence of disease-causing bacteria or parasites.

Toilet Training 201

While investigating the 'what' aspect of poop can reveal a lot about a person's health, considering the 'how' can also be quite useful. In fact, the way you position yourself on the toilet can affect the ease with which you eliminate. Sitting incorrectly can increase the risk of bowel and pelvic problems, especially constipation and hemorrhoids.

 As it turns out, virtually everyone living in the Western world is eliminating incorrectly.

While most of us consider the modern toilet a major upgrade over a hole in the ground, sitting with the legs at a 90-degree angle to the abdomen impedes the elimination process by kinking the colon. The human body is actually designed to eliminate by squatting, which allows the colon to remain open and the rectum to relax maximizing the ease and efficiency of elimination.

Evacuating the bowels more completely helps to prevent fecal stagnation and the accumulation of toxins in the intestinal tract. Societies in which people squat rather than sit have the lowest incidence of bowel disease.

Since the health benefits of squatting have become more widely recognized, there have been a number of products designed to promote proper potty posture. The simplest of these is a footstool; resting your feet on will allow you to use your toilet in a more natural, ergonomic position. The *Squatty Potty*® offers a space-saving design that allows you to tuck this stool around the base of your toilet when it's not in use.

How to Make Homemade Kombucha

Kombucha is a fermented tea made with water, tea, sugar, bacteria, and yeast. After a kombucha SCOBY sits in sweetened tea for 7-10 days, the result is a fermented, fizzy drink that's a fantastic source of probiotics (the good bacteria you want living in your gut).

SCOBY stands for symbiotic culture of bacteria and yeast. It's the slimy, jellyfish-like mushroom that works as a fermenting agent, turning what starts out as a sugar-sweetened tea into the perfect probiotic. You might be able to snag a spare SCOBY from one of your friends (a new one is generated with every batch so there's always one to share, shred and use as a dog food supplement, or compost. You can purchase one (typically online), or you can make your own from scratch using:

1. **A bottle of plain (not flavored) GT Dave's *Original Kombucha*.** Why GT Dave's? Because it reliably contains the live yeast strands that will serve as the starter culture for your home-grown SCOBY.

2. **Some black tea.** When you make future batches of kombucha, any caffeinated tea will work. But start with a black (like Oolong or Assam). Loose-leaf tea is more cost effective and tastes better than bags, but it has to be strained. Organic tea is always preferable.
3. **Unrefined, white sugar.** No other type of sugar will work. Don't be concerned about the calories, carbohydrates, or other downsides of white sugar in this case. It is being used to feed and nourish your SCOBY. By the end of the fermentation process, there will be little (if any) sugar left.
4. **Filtered water.** Start by bringing 2 cups water to boil in a small pot. Turn off the heat and add 1 bag or 1 teaspoon of tea and 3 tablespoons of sugar. Stir and cool completely before pouring into a glass quart jar (using a mesh strainer to filter leaves if necessary). Add 1 cup store-bought kombucha including any brownish strands from the bottle. Place the mixture in a crock or wide-mouth jar. Cover with a thin, breathable cloth secured with a rubber band and set away from direct sunlight (at a temperature between 70 and 80 degrees Fahrenheit. It takes two to four weeks to grow a SCOBY. You can take an occasional peek, but try not to disturb the jar. It will be ready to use when it's at least 1/4" thick and an opaque, white color.

To make your first batch of kombucha:

1. In a large pot, bring 14 cups (3 ½ quarts) of water, 4-5 tablespoons of tea, and 1 cup of sugar to boil then turn off the heat. Stir and allow to cool completely. Place your pot in a sink filled with cold water to speed the cooling process up. Don't keep the tea in a metal container overnight; it can take on a metallic taste.
2. In a gallon glass beverage dispenser or brewing crock, add your kombucha SCOBY and 2 cups of previously made kombucha (or liquid from your SCOBY making project). Pour the cooled tea on top through a mesh strainer.

3. Cover with a thin, breathable cloth secured with a rubber band and store at a temperature between 70 and 80 degrees Fahrenheit. Depending on where you live and how warm you keep your home, you may need to purchase a seed sprouting mat to keep the temperature constant during the winter months. Your ferment should be complete in about 7-10 days. It's perfectly okay if your SCOBY isn't floating at the top of your storage container; it will rise when you make subsequent batches.
4. After 7 days, start tasting your brew. If it still tastes sweet without any tartness, it's not quite done. Keep taking small samples every few days until the brew tastes tart with very little hint of any sweetness.
5. Transfer your brew into air-tight bottles using a funnel and enjoy. Juice-flavored kombucha should be kept in the refrigerator, but any extra from the batch can be left to go through a second ferment at room temperature (which adds a little extra fizz).
6. Have some fun browsing the internet for suggestions on how to flavor your probiotic homebrew!

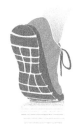

Obstacle Five

An Imbalanced Nervous System

The nervous system is one of the most incredible, yet inconspicuous, aspects of the human anatomy. It functions like a fine-tuned call center—accepting, analyzing, and disseminating information, carefully ensuring that accurate messages are sent to the correct recipients at exactly the right time. It's divided into two primary divisions: the central nervous system (CNS) and the peripheral nervous system (PNS).

The CNS consists of the brain and spinal cord. The PNS includes all the other nerves (that aren't a part of the CNS). The PNS can be broken down into two divisions: the sensory and the motor. The sensory division manages all tactile, auditory, olfactory, gustatory, and visual information. The motor division makes sure that the central nervous system's messages (nerve impulses) reach their intended recipient (the muscles). The motor division can be further separated into the somatic nervous system (SNS) and the autonomic nervous system (ANS).

The ANS is of vital importance because it constantly and consistently manages the body's ability to maintain internal homeostasis. It coordinates all of the body's unconscious activities including digestion, respiration, circulation, and elimination. In fact, the ANS influences every aspect of our physical and mental wellbeing. Even though we're not aware of its essential actions, the ANS and its three branches—the sympathetic, parasympathetic, and enteric—are always hard at work.

The sympathetic division of the autonomic nervous system activates the body's fight or flight response; the parasympathetic division, its rest and digest response. The actions of the enteric nervous system are confined to the gastrointestinal tract. Recent research has confirmed that the enteric nervous system, working in conjunction with the vagus nerve, acts as the body's second brain.

 The body is always listening and adapting to the messages it receives from the autonomic nervous system.

And it's this adaptability that largely determines an athlete's physical and mental aptitudes. The human nervous system is hardwired to react to stressors, and to become quiet in the absence of them. The symptoms of overtraining, poor performance, recurring injuries, frequent illness, and emotional burnout occur when an athlete's autonomic nervous system becomes over-stimulated and can no longer respond or adapt to the demands being placed upon it. ANS overload can also be expressed as an inability to shut down when it's appropriate. Women who seem to be stuck in a never-ending loop of non-stop activity are often struggling with a nervous system imbalance.

While the ANS plays a key role in managing the unconscious functions of the human body, the somatic nervous system is in charge of controlling and directing all muscular activity and movement. Just as the autonomic nervous system can become overloaded and malfunction, the somatic nervous system can become chronically over stimulated and incapable of switching off. When this happens, our muscles get tight; our bodies become rigid, and we become less flexible and physically adaptable.

 The body can only adapt to and benefit from the amount of stress it can process on a neurological level.

The specific amount of stress that serves an adaptive purpose can vary greatly from one woman to another. While most competitive athletes know that it's necessary to regularly reach or exceed their training stress threshold in order to elicit positive gains, there's another side of the equation to consider: training benefits can be diminished by as much as 40% if the body isn't allowed to recover completely after a hard effort. **More training is not always better, especially when it becomes a (maladaptive) form of chronic stress.**

Chronic Stress

Stress is an unavoidable aspect of modern life. And most of us are under a great deal of it, sometimes more than we realize. Our work and family lives are often stressful. Illnesses and injuries are always stressful. Even the activities we use to relieve stress (like training for and competing in a sport) can be stressful.

There are two main types of stress—acute and chronic. Acute stress is the immediate reaction to a threatening situation. Once the threat has passed, the function of our nervous system returns to normal with no damaging, long-term effects. In fact, there is some evidence to support the idea that small and regular amounts of acute stress can increase the brain's capacity for processing information faster and more efficiently.

Chronic stress is continuous and ongoing. And it can have a lasting, negative impact on both our physical and mental health. The body responds to acute stress by producing the short-lived hormones adrenaline and norepinephrine. It makes cortisol (in the adrenal glands) to facilitate our adaptation to long-term, chronic stress. Unfortunately, the body is not well-equipped to handle the sheer volume of chronic stress—or increased amounts of cortisol—that are now considered a 'normal' aspect of everyday life.

A chronically elevated cortisol level is extremely catabolic (destructive). It weakens the immune system, breaks down bone, muscle, and connective tissue, and interferes with thyroid hormone production. It promotes fat storage and speeds up the process of aging. Because a high cortisol level compromises both the quantity and quality of sleep, it will significantly reduce the body's ability to recover from an illness or injury.

Stress Resilience

Have you ever wondered why some women are more stress resistant than others? Why some thrive in high-pressure environments while others seem to self-destruct?

 It appears that the body's physiological stress response is governed by our perceptions.

Although there are certain events that almost all women experience as stressful, it's the subjective perception of these events—and the meaning we assign to them—that determines how much physiological stress we actually experience. Research has identified four key factors that influence our subjective perception of a stressor: the novelty and the unpredictability of the event, how threatening it is (to the body or the ego), and how much control we have over it.

The concept of perceived stress has some important implications. The most important of these is the notion that we can reduce the severity of our physiological response to a stressor by simply changing the way we think about it. In the field of psychology, this is known as 'reframing.'

Losing your job, for example, would be stressful; it's easy to imagine how your body might respond to that event. But if you viewed it as an opportunity to pursue a hidden passion or make a fresh start, it would be less likely to trigger a harmful stress response. It might even serve as a source of eustress or beneficial stress. Reframing gives us a measure of control over how we respond and adapt to life's stressful events. And strengthening our sense of control can enhance both our physical and mental wellbeing.

Stress and the Vagus Nerve

The vagus nerve is one of the most important, yet least familiar, parts of the autonomic central nervous system. The word *vagus* means wandering, which is the perfect way to describe this long, meandering bundle of sensory and motor neurons that extend from the brainstem to the neck, chest, and abdomen. A vagus nerve imbalance can lead to strained vocal chords, difficulty swallowing, hearing loss, an elevated heart rate, high blood pressure, constipation, and incontinence.

In addition to controlling and directing the activity of every major organ system in the body, the vagus nerve plays a critical role in mitigating the harmful effects of stress by activating the parasympathetic nervous response. Women with impaired vagal activity often suffer from depression, anxiety, and other mood disorders.

Women who have a strong vagal response (or healthy vagal tone) are characteristically resilient under stress. They can relax more quickly after a stressful event due to the strength of their parasympathetic nervous response. They also typically enjoy good digestion, a strong metabolism, and excellent overall mental and physical health.

Because life is hectic and demanding, however, the sympathetic nervous system is activated with greater frequency than the parasympathetic. So it often dominates our reflexive stress response. It is possible, however, to stimulate the vagus nerve, strengthening both its function and the body's ability to mitigate the harmful effects of stress.

Twelve Techniques for Increasing Vagal Tone

Chronic inflammation (the underlying cause of most illnesses and many injuries) is directly regulated by the brain, with the vagus nerve serving as the on/off switch. When the vagus nerve is stimulated, inflammation is reduced. Implementing just one or two of the following techniques on a regular basis will strengthen the vagus nerve, expanding the body's potential for optimal health, performance, and recovery.

1. **Practice mindful breathing.** Deep, rhythmic breathing is one of the most powerful ways to stimulate the vagus nerve. While the use of breathing techniques is a relatively new concept in the West, Eastern medicine has been incorporating them for millennia. It is now widely accepted that deep breathing plays an important role in supporting the body's ability to achieve and maintain physiological balance.

   We all have experienced the benefits of taking several deep breaths to calm down prior to the start of an event or during a period of emotional distress. Deep breathing essentially 'kick starts' the body's parasympathetic response by activating the vagus nerve. It turns out that the benefits of deep breathing are even greater when practiced on a regular basis.

   Mindful breathing doesn't require any extra time or effort, but it does demand some focused attention. It's important to breathe in fully, allowing your belly to relax and expand. When breathing out, the opposite should happen—the belly should contract inward, pushing the last remnants of air out of the lungs. The more your belly expands and contracts, the deeper your breathing will become. Taking five or six deep breaths a minute is a very achievable goal for most women.

2. **Do some yoga.** Yoga has been shown to improve both vagal tone and parasympathetic activity, especially when combined with mindful breathing. Research indicates that women who do yoga regularly experience less anxiety and have a more positive outlook on life. In addition to stimulating the vagus nerve, the practice of yoga has been shown to raise levels of gamma-aminobutyric acid or GABA, which has a natural, calming effect on the brain.

3. **Consider the use of a probiotic supplement.** The vagus nerve is constantly sending information about the status of the body's internal organs to the brain. We now know that the health of our intestinal microbiome can have a profound effect on how well the vagus nerve does its job. Eating a healthy, balanced diet that

includes fermented foods will enhance the health of the microbiome and support the vagus nerve's ability to communicate more clearly.

Studies also suggest that the use of probiotic supplements will improve the body's microbiome and support a healthy parasympathetic response. In fact, recent research has shown them to be an effective treatment for both anxiety disorders and post-traumatic stress syndrome or PTSD. Avoiding the unnecessary use of antibiotics and limiting both sugar and alcohol intake will be helpful, too.

4. **Take a balanced approach to exercise.** We all know that physical activity is good for the mind and body. But when it comes to stimulating the vagus nerve, it's important to make sure that the amount and intensity of exercise doesn't exceed a 'tonic' level.

   While competitive athletes are occasionally required to push the boundaries of their physical limitations, pursuing activities that can be done at a comfortable level of exertion will do more to improve the health of the vagus nerve. Finding a balance between goal-oriented workouts and joyful movement can make the mind and body stronger and more stress-resistant.

5. **Get a massage.** Neck, foot, and full-body pressure massage can stimulate the vagus nerve, supporting growth, repair, and recovery. In fact, massage is often used to help underweight infants gain weight because it stimulates the vagus nerve.

6. **Chill out.** Studies show that when the body adjusts to cold, its parasympathetic system switches on. So short-term cold exposure will stimulate vagal activity. The simplest way to start? Splash a little cold water on your face. Submerging your face in cold water for a short period of time would be a next step. Those who are motivated can graduate to taking a brief, cold shower.

7. **Sing a song or listen to music.** Humming, chanting, and singing all activate the vagus nerve. Listening to music can get the job done,

too. We enjoy music because it stirs our emotions and leaves us with a heightened sense of wellbeing. These positive feelings are inextricably linked to vagal activation.

8. **Laugh a lot.** As the saying goes, "Laughter is the best medicine." In fact, numerous studies have proven that it's possible to laugh your way to better health since it stimulates and strengthens the vagus nerve. It enhances cognitive function, protects against heart disease, encourages the release of feel-good endorphins, and supports the production of nitric oxide (which improves oxygen delivery).

9. **Pray or meditate.** Prayer and meditation have both been shown to increase vagal tone. Prayer slows and deepens breathing, which stimulates the vagus nerve and strengthens cardiovascular health. One study showed that reciting the rosary (a Catholic prayer practice) increased vagal activity and improved diastolic blood pressure.

   Studies have shown that meditation can also improve the function of the vagus nerve, although it seems to be more effective when the process includes compassionate thoughts. Repeating phrases like "may you feel safe" or "may you be happy" amplify the positive emotional effects of meditating by encouraging a greater sense of connectedness to others. Combining meditation with social connection improves vagal tone, increasing our sense of joy, serenity, and compassion.

10. **Practice giving.** Most women find giving to others an inherently enjoyable practice. It turns out that there's a physiological reason why. Giving our time, attention, or resources to another stimulates the vagus nerve. Researchers believe that a branch of our nervous system evolved to reinforce our giving behavior with positive physical and psychological benefits, which probably played a role in guaranteeing the survival of our species.

11. **Sleep or rest on your right side.** Studies have found that sleeping or lying on the right side encourages the highest level of vagal activation; lying on the back, the lowest.
12. **Give it a gargle.** Gargling activates the vagus nerve and stimulates the gastrointestinal tract (improving digestion). Before you swallow water, give it an occasional gargle first.

Heart Rate Variability, Vagal Tone, and Recovery Status

The condition of your vagus nerve can be measured by tracking certain biological processes such as your heart rate, breathing rate, and heart rate variability (HRV). The use of HRV involves measuring the time gaps between heart beats. This variability is a result of the allostatic (adaptive) processes of the body.

Although it may sound counter-intuitive, the more variability there is, the higher your vagal tone, stress resilience, and recovery capacity. With no input from the autonomic nervous system, a healthy heart contracts at an intrinsic rate of about 100 beats per minute. Parasympathetic regulation lowers the heart rate from its intrinsic level, giving more room for variability between beats. Sympathetic regulation does just the opposite; it elevates the heart rate leaving less room for variability.

A high HRV score means that your body is doing a good job of adapting to the levels of mental and physical stress it's being exposed to. It also correlates with a larger aerobic capacity and an increased readiness to train hard with a reduced risk of illness or injury. As a result, it can be used as a fitness barometer to accurately predict an athlete's performance and recovery potential.

When it comes to our training, we use heart rate monitors and power meters; we time our intervals in the pool and at the track. We use lots of different metrics for measuring our performance, but we don't pay nearly enough attention to the quantity and quality of our recovery.

Since rest is when our bodies have the opportunity to repair, regenerate, and make positive performance gains, it makes sense to place some emphasis on measuring our recovery efforts, too. But subjectively relying on intuition or how we feel isn't always accurate. Heart rate variability is an easy-to-use tool that can objectively assess the state of your autonomic nervous system and, as a result, your training readiness and recovery status.

When the body is in a state of sympathetic dominance, its ability to recover is impaired. Ideally, the recovering athlete should pursue relaxing activities that promote parasympathetic dominance, which is when our heart and breathing rates slow. Because we don't need to run, fight, or hide, the body directs blood flow away from the skeletal muscles and to the organs. We digest our food. We make hormones. We repair our cells. We gain strength. Our body is in a state of relaxation, and this relaxation promotes recovery. **The more time we spend in a state of parasympathetic dominance, the healthier we become.**

Reframing Recovery

The topic of overtraining gets a lot of attention—and for good reason. If pushed too hard and too far for too long, the body will stop responding positively to training stress. However, the concept of 'under-recovering' merits equal time and attention. In the vast majority of cases, it isn't an athlete's training that's the problem; it's her lack of recovery.

 If you spend any time using social media, you probably have access to more than enough training tips. Advice on how, when, and why you should be recovering is a lot less readily available.

This is unfortunate because we don't make performance gains during exercise; we make them during rest.

While the right kind of stress can lead to adaptive, performance-enhancing outcomes, the wrong kind can be physically and mentally debilitating. If your total stress load is too high, your body will respond by creating more cortisol and less dopamine, which contributes to delayed or incomplete recovery from exercise, illness, and/or injury.

Planned periods of recovery give the body a regular opportunity to dedicate its resources to positive adaptations. While at rest, the vascular network can expand (increasing oxygen delivery) and the nervous system can become more efficient at contracting and relaxing the muscles. On a cellular level, the mitochondria (the energy production centers of the cell) are given the chance to multiply for improved energy production.

Regular recovery is good for the mental aspect of an athlete's performance, too. It can help prevent burnout by maintaining motivation. Mental fatigue can be as detrimental to an athlete's health and performance as physical fatigue. A rest day can help recharge the mind, body, and spirit.

Taking a rest day doesn't make you weak, it makes you strong.

While you probably already have some fairly well-defined training goals, consider setting some specific recovery goals, too. And remember: a rest day doesn't necessarily have to mean a day without any exercise (although there is a time and a place for this). Research has consistently shown that active recovery is much more beneficial than putting a hard stop to all physical activity. Taking a walk, going for an easy bike ride, working on your swim technique, or participating in a yoga class are just a few of the things you can do on your next 'day off.'

Tips for Managing and Reducing Stress

Avoiding (or at least reducing) stress should become a top priority for every athlete, regardless of her competitive aspirations. While there's no one-size-fits-all formula for achieving a lower stress level, here are some helpful tips:

1. **Move slowly.** To counterbalance the physiological stress of hard, physical effort, the body needs to move slowly. Do some kind of relaxing activity at least twice a week that will give your body the opportunity to recharge—both physically and mentally.

   Remember: the body doesn't respond well to periods of complete inactivity. If you have a job that requires lots of sitting, get up and move away from your desk at regular intervals. Try to stand up or change positions at your desk once every 20 minutes, and walk for five to 10 minutes every hour (preferably outside if the logistics and weather permit). Recent research shows that no amount of exercise or type of physical activity will overcome the negative physiological effects of a sedentary day.

2. **Vary the type and intensity of your workouts.** If you're only doing long, slow distance, you're only using and training one of the body's energy systems. You're also missing out on an opportunity to make your body (and mind) more stress-resistant. To optimize your body's capacity for stress, consider adding some short-burst interval training (high-intensity activity repeats combined with intermittent recovery periods). This specific type of high-intensity interval training mimics the stress response—short periods of increased heart rate, breathing, and muscle use followed by unstructured periods of recovery.

   There is a direct connection between training the heart to recover after an exercise-induced stress and getting it to recover after an episode of life stress. In fact, training the body to recover from any type of stress—physical, mental, or emotional—improves the body's ability to adapt on both a physiological and neurological level. Short-burst interval training improves the body's ability to recover from stress more quickly and efficiently. It also raises the 'trigger point' at which the body decides what is or isn't stressful. Over time, the body becomes conditioned to accept a greater stress load without responding to it.

3. **Stay hydrated.** Even mild dehydration can significantly impair the body's ability to repair and recover. Keep a glass container or stainless steel water bottle with you and sip water throughout the day. There are a range of water recommendations, but the easiest way to assess how you're doing is to check your urine color. Consistently clear is the goal.

4. **Get at least 20 minutes of exposure to sunlight daily.** Exposure to sunlight is thought to increase the brain's release of serotonin—the mood-boosting neurochemical that can improve your ability to stay calm, focused, and stress-free. Sunlight is also necessary for the production of vitamin D3 and nitric oxide, which both keep stress hormone levels in check.

5. **Make time for yourself every day.** Take a walk in the woods. Listen to some calming music, watch your favorite sit-com, read a book, invite a friend over for a glass of wine or a cup of coffee. If you're spiritual, dedicate a portion of each day to practicing your faith. Five to 10 minutes of silence a day can make you significantly more stress-hardy.

6. **Sleep deep.** When it comes to maximizing the body's ability to offload accumulated stress, nothing is more powerful than a good night's sleep. In fact, this is the only window of opportunity the body has to dedicate 100% of its resources to repair and restoration. Got stress? Get some sleep.

Foods and Supplements for Buffering Stress

Although we can't see or feel it happening, stress affects the body by depleting its existing stores of essential vitamins and minerals—and by interfering with the efficiency of their initial absorption during digestion. Because they are used in the production of stress-related hormones and neurotransmitters, these micronutrients are diverted from the more constructive jobs they could (and should) otherwise be doing inside the body.

A growing body of research supports the use of certain adaptogenic herbs or adaptogens to buffer the harmful effects of stress.

The use of adaptogens is quite common in the practice of phytotherapy—the use of plant-derived medications in the prevention and treatment of disease. Adaptogenic herbs have long been shown to be effective in reducing stress by naturally lowering cortisol.

Some of the most popular adaptogens include ashwagandha, astragalus, licorice, Asian and Siberian ginseng roots; rhodiola, holy basil, and schisandra. If you lead a high-stress life, there may be a place for herbal supplementation. But eating a varied diet that includes whole, unprocessed foods that are rich in the right stress-buffering vitamins and minerals should be the first place to start.

As a group, the B vitamins are known for their ability to improve mood, calm the nervous system, and increase stress tolerance.

There are eight B vitamins, some of which can be obtained from both plant and animal foods. Others are found mainly in plants (such as vitamin B9) or exclusively in animal foods (vitamin B12). Since no single food can offer all of the B vitamins, it's important to eat a wide variety of both plant and animal-based foods.

Vitamin C is the most widely used supplement because of its many benefits, which include increased stress resilience.

Since vitamin C controls the formation of the stress hormone cortisol, it promotes stress tolerance and supports the body's ability to bounce back faster from a stressful event. It's also an essential cofactor in the production of soothing serotonin. All animals—except humans—can make their own supply of vitamin C. For this reason, we need to source it from foods and/or supplements.

In general, fruits are the best dietary source of vitamin C. Citrus fruits, strawberries, and tropical fruits like pineapple, papaya, and kiwi lead the list. The best vegetable sources are peppers of all kinds, tomatoes, and cruciferous vegetables (broccoli, Brussels sprouts, cauliflower, and kale). Keep in mind that these vegetable sources typically contain less than 100 mg of vitamin C per serving. If you have been searching for a high-quality supplement, I can recommend either Nutrigold *Organic Vitamin C* or Pure Radiance *Natural Vitamin C Powder*. Both of these non-synthetic, botanically derived products can be found on Amazon.

Magnesium is often called the 'master mineral' because it assists in more than 600 different metabolic functions.

 There's a direct correlation between low magnesium and the body's susceptibility to stress. So optimizing your magnesium level is one of the most important things you can do to become more stress-resistant.

One way magnesium neutralizes stress is by binding to and stimulating gamma-aminobutyric acid (GABA) receptors in the brain. Since GABA calms an overstimulated brain, classic signs of a deficiency include racing thoughts (especially while trying to fall asleep at night) and feeling easily overwhelmed. When GABA is low, it becomes difficult or impossible to relax.

The top food sources of magnesium include nuts and seeds, spinach, black beans, avocado, non-glutinous grains, and fermented soy. Keep in mind that legumes, seeds, and grains also contain phytates which inhibit the absorption of many minerals, including magnesium. This is one of the reasons why it's difficult to get enough magnesium from food alone.

Another reason is that much of our food is grown in magnesium-depleted soils, even if it's organic. And there are more than 200 different medications that can interfere with magnesium absorption. The biggest culprits include acid blockers, laxatives, diuretics, and blood pressure medications.

If you decide to supplement, I recommend using a form of magnesium called Magtein™, which can be found in a variety of different products. I personally use Life Extension *NeuroMag* every night. This particular product has been shown to increase brain magnesium levels for improved cognition, sleep, and mood; and for combating a variety of other conditions linked to chronic stress and accelerated aging.

Zinc is another mineral required for good overall health and mental wellbeing because it plays a vital role in modulating the body's stress response. Zinc supports the production and action of GABA (the anti-anxiety hormone). Along with vitamin B6, it's a cofactor in the production of serotonin. Zinc is frequently used as a supportive nutrient in the treatment of depression.

It's very important to understand that zinc has an inverse relationship with copper. It's not just the total amount of zinc you take in, but the balance between zinc and copper that contributes to the body's capacity for managing stress and anxiety.

 Women who experience anxiety and poor vagal tone often have an elevated level of copper and a low level of zinc.

Excess copper heightens the body's stress response by blocking GABA and increasing the production of epinephrine and norepinephrine— the acute stress hormones.

The naturally occurring copper we consume in our food is generally not a problem since can be processed and eliminated by the liver. It's the *inorganic* (not from a plant or animal) copper found in water pipes, cookware, medications, and even multivitamin supplements that collectively contribute to an excess. Once it enters the bloodstream, copper can cross the blood-brain barrier where it can contribute to the onset of neurodegenerative disease, an umbrella term for a range of conditions which negatively affect neurological function.

Ironically, the foods highest in zinc are also highest in copper—oysters, crab, beef, legumes, and nuts. So eating zinc-rich foods won't be the best strategy for achieving a healthy zinc-copper balance; it's better to use a zinc supplement. As a general rule, your dietary intake of zinc to copper should remain in a ratio of roughly 10:1.

A Closer Look at the B Vitamins

Natural health practitioners have been promoting the use of the B vitamins as a stress and anxiety remedy for years. These essential nutrients also play a fundamental role in keeping our bodies running smoothly and efficiently by helping us convert food into fuel.

While many of them work in tandem, each of the eight B vitamins also has its own specific benefits:

- **Vitamin B1** (thiamine) strengthens the immune system, helps regulate blood sugar, and improves the body's capacity for stress resilience. Best sources are non-glutinous, 'ancient' grains; meat, fish, legumes, seeds, and nuts.
- **Vitamin B2** (riboflavin) helps break down proteins, fats, and carbohydrates. It plays a particularly vital role in maintaining the body's energy supply by aiding the conversion of carbohydrates into adenosine triphosphate or ATP (the body's basic energy currency). Best sources are eggs, meat, organ meats, full-fat dairy products, and green vegetables.

- **Vitamin B3** (niacin) suppresses chronic inflammation, which is caused or worsened by stress. Best sources are meat, fish, poultry, mushrooms, and peanuts.
- **Vitamin B5** (pantothenic acid) is one of the most important vitamins for human life. It's necessary for making blood cells, and balancing blood sugar. Best sources are meat, dairy, eggs, legumes, mushrooms, avocados, broccoli, and sweet potatoes.
- **Vitamin B6** (pyridoxine) is utilized in the synthesis of the stress hormones epinephrine and norepinephrine, which leaves less for its other function—supporting the production of the feel-good neurotransmitters GABA, serotonin, and dopamine. Best sources are poultry, fish, organ meats, potatoes, starchy vegetables, and non-citrus fruits.
- **Vitamin B7** (biotin) supports healthy neurological function and metabolism; and it assists in creating a wide variety of enzymes. It is sometimes referred to as 'vitamin H' because it provides particularly nourishing benefits to the hair. Best sources are meat, fish, poultry, eggs, and full-fat dairy products.
- **Vitamin B9** (folate or folic acid) supports healthy adrenal and brain function; it helps calm the nervous system and boost metabolism. Best sources are green leafy vegetables, liver, yeast, black-eyed peas, and Brussels sprouts.
- **Vitamin B12** (cobalamin) assists the body in many ways, but it's primarily used to support healthy nerve cell function and red blood cell formation. Best sources are clams, liver, and red meat.

If you decide to supplement with B vitamins, look for a food-based formula such as New Chapter's *Coenzyme B Complex* or Pure Synergy's *Super-B Complex*.

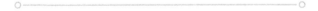

The Need for Deep Sleep

One of the most powerful, yet most under-utilized, strategies for re-balancing and re-booting the nervous system is sleep. Unfortunately, it's often the first trade-off a time-poor athlete makes. And popular sayings like, "I'll sleep when I'm dead" reinforce the idea that sleep is unimportant.

Because athletes are continually exposed to physical and psychological stressors, both the quantity and the quality of their sleep should be considered essential recovery variables. Sleep is not only when the muscles, tissues, and cells have their biggest window of opportunity to repair and rebuild, it's when cognitive and neurological function is restored.

 The central nervous system is the information highway of the body. Sleep is what keeps its lanes and interchanges functioning efficiently.

Without an adequate amount of sleep, road signs end up facing the wrong way; exits and on ramps are randomly shut down. A lack of quality sleep will disrupt the flow of information throughout the entire body.

During sleep, pathways form between nerve cells (neurons) in your brain that help you remember any new information you've learned. For this reason, sleep deprivation interferes with both memory and recall. And it can negatively affect your ability to focus and concentrate. A lack of sleep can make you feel more impatient and prone to mood swings. It compromises decision-making skills and cripples the creative process. In addition, the predictability and reliability of the signals your nervous system sends to the rest of the body may also be compromised, diminishing motor coordination and increasing the risk of an injury or accident.

The next time your busy schedule forces you to make a choice between sleeping a few extra hours and getting a training session in, perform a cost/benefit analysis to see what the risk/reward ratio really is.

Of course, no two athletes will require the same amount of sleep. The exact number of hours you need depends on your genes, diet, stress level, training schedule, and age (among other things). Most active women need a minimum of eight hours a night. But consider this: Michelle Wie feels and performs her best with at least 12 hours of sleep. Lindsey Vonn, Venus Williams, and Maria Sharapova all strive for a minimum of 10.

Casey Smith, the Head Athletic Trainer of the Dallas Mavericks, has said, "If you told an athlete you had a treatment that would reduce the chemicals associated with stress, that would naturally increase human growth hormone, that enhances recovery rate, that improves performance, they would all do it. Sleep does all of those things."

What does the research say about athletes who don't get enough sleep?

They have significantly slower reaction times, higher injury rates, and weaker immune systems. They are more likely to be forgetful, depressed, stressed, anxious, and angry. Without enough sleep, we can't effectively regulate our emotions, benefit fully from our training, or recover quickly from an illness or injury.

Research also indicates that sleeping less than eight hours a night can interfere with our circadian rhythm or internal 'body clock' that regulates a multitude of physiological processes. When a woman's circadian rhythm is disrupted, her physical and mental health can both be compromised.

Sunrise, Sunset

For billions of years, the evolution of earth's life forms has been driven by the consistent rising and setting of the sun. This same circadian rhythm is what continues to dictate our sleeping patterns and the timing of important, hormonal secretions.

When the sun sets, for example, the sleep hormone melatonin is released into the bloodstream, activating a process referred to as dim light melatonin onset or DLMO. When the sun rises, our serotonin level increases so that we can wake feeling refreshed.

A growing body of research confirms the adverse effects a disrupted circadian rhythm can have on both our physical and mental health.

> It's important to recognize, however, that a woman's circadian rhythm—and sleep time preferences—can be influenced by her *chronotype.*

There's a pervasive belief that early risers are somehow superior to those who stay up and wake up late. But 'night owls' are just as healthy, focused, and productive as 'early birds.' They simply run on a different time schedule.

While you probably already know if you're a morning or night person, Dr. Michael Breus, sleep expert and author of *The Power of When,* has taken the analysis of circadian rhythms one step further by identifying four distinctly different chronotypes, associating each with an animal whose sleep/wake habits mirror them most accurately:

- **The Bear.** The most common chronotype (50-55% of the total population) is the Bear with a sleep/wake cycle that follows the sun. Bears typically don't suffer from sleeping disorders and tend to feel most prepared for tackling intense tasks mid-morning. They do, however, tend to experience a dip in energy during the mid-afternoon. Bears enjoy a relatively steady energy pattern and can be productive all day, as long as they don't try to push through the mid-afternoon rest period they need. Bears tend to be outgoing, friendly, and highly efficient.
- **The Lion.** About 15% of us are Lions, the quintessential early risers that are often viewed as overachievers. They wake up organized, energized, and ready to roar. They might not even think about reaching for their morning cup of coffee until just before lunch, by which time most of their productive hours have passed. Because of their intense, action-packed mornings, Lions tend to turn in early.
- **The Wolf.** Another 15% of us are Wolves, who exist on the nocturnal end of the spectrum. Since their days start later, Wolves tend to be more productive when the rest of the world is already winding down. And they tend to be creative types—writers, artists, and coders. In fact, the creative areas of the Wolf's brain light up when the sun goes down. More often than not, Wolf types tend toward introversion and crave time alone.
- **The Dolphin.** Dolphins represent the remaining 10% of the population that may or may not have a regular sleep routine.

Dolphins struggle to fall (and stay) asleep, so they often struggle with insomnia and other sleep-related disorders. Dolphins tend to be extremely intelligent and have perfectionistic tendencies, which is why many ruminate over the day's perceived failures when they lie down to sleep at night. Due to their strong sense of loyalty, Dolphins make trustworthy friends.

 While it is possible to shift your sleep/wake times to accommodate early-morning training sessions, your performance gains may be greater when you can work with your body's innate programming.

"I always tell people you can't mess with mother nature. This is genetically predetermined. This isn't something that you just have a preference for. It's actually the PER3 gene that determines your sleep drive, and then your circadian rhythms," explains Breus.

Regardless of what chronotype you are, getting enough sleep is an absolute essential for optimal female health and performance.

One indicator you can use to assess whether or not you are getting enough sleep is your dream state. It's a positive sign if you wake with the feeling that you were dreaming the entire night. Dreams begin during the latter portion of each phase of your nightly sleep cycle.

Although we aren't aware of it, the brain is quite active during sleep. Instead of responding to the external stimuli it processes during the time we're awake, however, it shifts to processing countless bits of internal information as we sleep. Throughout the course of any given night, it drifts in and out of different sleep stages. Stage one, for example, marks the initial transition into sleep. Stage two accounts for about 50% of our total sleep time. This is when the brain sorts through information and solidifies learning, uploading items that are later processed for long-term memory storage. Most of sleep's restorative benefits occur during stage three. This slow-wave stage is predominant during the earlier periods of sleep.

After sleeping anywhere from 70 to 100 minutes, we enter REM (rapid eye movement) sleep. This dream-dominated stage accounts for about 20% of our total sleep time. During REM, the brain sorts and sifts through emotional experiences and stressful events while placing all the information it collected during stage two into long-term storage.

We move through several sleep cycles each night, each lasting about 90 minutes. Experiencing more complete sleep cycles results in more REM or dream sleep. One full night of sleep can be divided into three, distinctly different time periods: the first is characterized by more deep sleep, the last by more REM sleep, and the middle is a relatively even mix of the other two.

Female Hormones and Sleep Disturbances

A common complaint among many women (especially those who are postmenopausal) is that they just can't sleep, no matter what they do. Low hormone levels are largely to blame. As estrogen and progesterone decrease after menopause, the likelihood of sleep disturbances increase.

Estrogen regulates the ANS by increasing both serotonin and dopamine. These neurotransmitters enhance the quantity and quality of sleep by making it easier for a woman to fall asleep and spend more time in REM sleep (which restores the central nervous system and promotes healthy brain chemistry balance). They reduce periods of wakefulness by keeping cortisol levels in check.

With less estrogen, the sympathetic system becomes dominant allowing cortisol to spike more easily at night in response to noise or light. Low progesterone levels disrupt melatonin production and core temperature regulation, both of which contribute to the incidence of night sweats and poor sleep.

Practicing Good Sleep Hygiene

Sleep hygiene—a set of practices that promote high-quality sleep—is becoming a bit of a 'buzzword' these days. But what, exactly, does it entail?

Perhaps the most basic tenet of sleep hygiene is simply to sleep enough. While the average woman needs a minimum of eight hours of sleep each night, female athletes will likely need more. Those who are injured or ill will definitely need more.

Learning to embrace the dark is another essential sleep hygiene habit to adopt. While watching TV or reading from a tablet might seem like a great way to relax and unwind at night, the artificial light that these devices emit can interfere with your natural circadian rhythm. This makes you more prone to the nervous system imbalances that ultimately increase the incidence of hormonal and metabolic dysfunction.

Electronics of all kinds emit blue light. And the bluer the light, the higher it registers on the Kelvin temperature scale. As a reference point, ultraviolet sunlight at noon measures 5,500K; most computer monitors, 6,500K. Such intense exposure causes a spike in cortisol which not only inhibits sleep, but increases hunger, causes sugar cravings, and promotes insulin production (which encourages fat storage while you sleep).

If you struggle with sleep issues, consider taking steps to minimize your exposure to blue light after the sun sets. Use more low-temperature light (in the red-orange-yellow spectrum), which will not interfere with the natural release of melatonin into your system. If exposure to blue light is unavoidable, consider purchasing a pair of yellow-tinted sunglasses (which will filter out blue light). You can also download a free program called *Flux* which synchronizes the color temperature of your screen to the ambient light in your environment, effectively reducing your blue light exposure.

Other good sleep hygiene habits include:

- **Implementing consistent bed and wake times.**
- **Allowing yourself a few extra minutes for a more gentle awakening.** Stretch, read for a few minutes, set an intention for the day, or practice some diaphragmatic breathing instead of immediately springing up and into action. If you use an alarm, opt for a calming, nature-inspired sound rather than a harsh blast or beep.
- **Creating a comfortable and organized sleeping environment and using the bedroom only for sleep.** Remove any work materials and eliminate clutter like loose clothing, newspapers, or magazines. The bedroom should be cool (between 60 and 65 degrees Fahrenheit) for optimal sleep. Consider using ear plugs, a white noise app, or a fan in order to overcome any ambient noise issues; and think about buying heavy, blackout curtains, room-darkening blinds, or an eye mask so that you can sleep in complete darkness.

- **Avoiding refined, high-carbohydrate foods,** especially in the evening. They can result in unwanted, insulin-spiking consequences during sleep.

Supplements and Foods for Sleep

Valerian root is a common herbal remedy that has been used in traditional medicine to promote relaxation and sleep for at least 2,000 years. A number of studies have found that it reduces both the amount of time it takes to fall asleep and that required to enter a state of deep sleep. But keep in mind that about one in every 10 women actually feel energized by the use of valerian. Taking too much of it can also be overstimulating.

In addition to cuing the onset of sleep, melatonin serves to regulate our circadian rhythms and sleep/wake cycles. The body begins to manufacture melatonin somewhere between three and four months of life (when a baby's ability to sleep through the night becomes more common). Its production peaks between the ages of two and three then drops slightly to a plateau that lasts throughout early adulthood. Melatonin secretion does, however, decline with age. At the age of 70, most adults produce only a quarter of the melatonin they did at the age of 20.

Several placebo-controlled studies have shown that the use of a melatonin supplement can significantly improve the onset, quality, and quantity of sleep. A dose of one to five milligrams of melatonin taken about 45 minutes before bed is the standard recommendation. Because its efficacy can be compromised by the digestive process, sublingual sprays (which are directly absorbed into the bloodstream) are generally more effective than tablets or lozenges.

Recent studies have also supported the sleep-enhancing effects of tart cherries and cherry juice. A study by Russel Reiter of the University of Texas Health Science Center found that cherries contain a significant amount of melatonin. Some women find that drinking a few ounces of tart cherry juice a half hour to 45 minutes before bed helps them fall asleep faster and stay asleep longer.

 While this may come as a surprise, there's some strong evidence to support the idea that having a correctly constructed bedtime snack will aid and enhance sleep.

Conventional wisdom maintains that we shouldn't eat after a certain time at night. And this advice is partially sound. There are certain foods that tend to interfere with or reduce the quality of sleep. Sugar, alcohol, spicy foods, fatty foods, and caffeine are all repeat offenders.

The most common argument waged against the bedtime snack is that it provides unnecessary calories since the body doesn't need energy during sleep. If it were just about calories, then this argument might be valid. But the body's metabolic process is driven by so much more than calories. **And as you know by now, it's the quality (nutrient density) not the quantity of food that matters most.** Macronutrient (and micronutrient) ratios matter, too. And your metabolism doesn't close up shop just because you're sleeping. With your brain still working and vital processes still functioning, your blood sugar still needs to be stable.

Very active (or chronically stressed) women often sleep better when they bring their blood sugar level slightly back up 15 to 30 minutes before heading to bed. Combining small and relatively equal amounts of a more complex carbohydrate and a healthy fat can sometimes work wonders. While the carbohydrate elevates blood sugar, the fat slows and stabilizes the assimilation of nutrients throughout the night.

Your snack strategy can (and should) be fairly simple—a handful of fresh berries eaten with about the same amount of nuts or topped with a tablespoon of unsweetened heavy (or full-fat coconut) cream; half of a small sweet potato topped with a generous amount of butter and a dash of cinnamon; half of a small banana with two tablespoons of peanut butter. As an upgraded alternative to the age-old sleep remedy of a glass of warm milk, try a few ounces of coconut milk heated and blended with a few teaspoons of almond butter and raw honey. The options are almost endless.

Why no protein? Because it can cause sleep disturbances for many women. The right amounts of high-quality protein are a dietary staple during the day, but not at night when the goal is to optimize sleep. In addition to being the most energy-intensive macronutrient to digest, protein contains the amino acid tyrosine which increases conscious brain activity.

Is Coffee Bad for the Nervous System?

If you love coffee, you're not alone. Americans drink almost three million cups of it a day. So it's somewhat comforting to know that there are several confirmed benefits associated with its consumption. In fact, a number of research studies show that drinking coffee in moderation can prevent certain cancers, stroke, and diabetes; Parkinson's, Alzheimer's, and cardiovascular disease; gout, gallstones, and depression. It can protect against antibiotic-resistant bacterial infections and liver disease. It can even reduce muscle soreness after a workout. Many of these effects are attributed to the polyphenols (the beneficial plant-based compounds that give coffee its bitter taste), antioxidants, and other bioactive compounds found in coffee (including some with insulin-sensitizing and anti-inflammatory properties).

Coffee also contains caffeine, which has proven benefits—for some. Generally speaking, caffeine has an anti-inflammatory effect inside the body. And if you're one of those women who feels more productive and energized after a morning latte, then your brain is experiencing the positive benefits of increased energy metabolism. But not everyone reacts to caffeine in a positive way.

About a decade ago, Dr. Ahmed El-Sohemy, a professor in the department of nutritional sciences at the University of Toronto became interested in studying the different ways people respond to coffee. Some feel jittery and anxious while others feel focused and alert. He quickly zeroed in on a particular gene (CYP1A2) that determines how quickly the body breaks down caffeine.

One variant of the gene causes the liver to metabolize caffeine quickly. Women who inherit two copies of the 'fast' variant are known as *fast metabolizers*. Their bodies metabolize caffeine about four times more quickly than the slow metabolizers who inherit one or more copies of the 'slow' variant. About 50% of the population has a variant in the CYP1A2 gene that slows down the body's ability to process caffeine.

Because caffeine hangs around a lot longer in the system of a slow metabolizer, it's more likely to cause negative side effects like insomnia, anxiety, and an upset stomach. There is also evidence that slow metabolizers (who drink large amounts of coffee) are more prone to non-fatal heart attacks and/or high blood pressure.

Although the long-standing assumption is that caffeine enhances sports performance, research done by Dr. Christopher Womack, a professor of kinesiology at James Madison University, suggests that athletes who are fast metabolizers will reap greater benefits than the slow. The more rapid metabolism of caffeine is necessary to heighten the adaptive response of the sympathetic nervous system, improving athletic performance.

But too much of a good thing can be a bad thing, even for fast metabolizers. Excessive coffee intake can cause gastrointestinal discomfort, a racing heart, and disrupted sleep when it over stimulates the autonomic nervous system. Evidence also suggests that too much coffee can negatively affect a woman's estrogen levels, raise her blood pressure, and trigger the excessive release of stress hormones.

As a general recommendation, limit your daily intake of caffeinated coffee to no more than two cups, preferably before 2:00 p.m. And consider reframing coffee as a type of nutrient support.

Be selective in the type of coffee you choose, always opting for high-quality (organic, single-origin, and mold-free beans) over quantity. Too much caffeine can stress the adrenals, cause dehydration, and lead to other unpleasant side effects ranging from acid reflux to anxiety.

If you need to curb your coffee habit, drink some warm water before your first cup. And try to avoid having coffee on a completely empty stomach; its acidity can adversely affect the lining of your stomach and intestines. When consumed after a meal, coffee acts as a natural digestive aid.

What about tea? While the caffeine in tea and coffee are technically identical, they differ in three ways:

1. There is significantly less caffeine in the average cup of tea, especially green and white teas and any tea variety that's brewed for a shorter time at a cooler temperature.
2. L-theanine, an amino acid found only in tea, reduces stress and promotes relaxation. It works with caffeine in a synergistic way to calm the body without reducing alertness.
3. The high levels of antioxidants found in tea slow the absorption of its caffeine which results in a gentler introduction of the chemical into the system and a longer period of alertness without a resulting 'crash' at the end.

There are still some outstanding questions about caffeine that haven't been completely answered. And these may have to do with other genetic variants or physiological differences that are not yet fully understood. Caffeine consumed in the afternoon or evening significantly disrupts sleep in some fast metabolizers, but not in others. Some slow metabolizers might be adversely affected by caffeine while others experience a gradual and long-lasting boost from their morning brew. Can these inconsistencies be attributed to a woman's dietary choices? Her stress level? Her ancestry? The number of hours she sleeps?

 We don't have all the answers. But we do know enough to stop asking the question, "Is coffee good or bad?" And to ask instead, "Is coffee good or bad for me?"

If you want an answer to this question without doing any genetic testing, gradually reduce your intake of all caffeinated beverages until you can remain off them entirely for at least 21 days. Then add them back into your diet, paying close attention to how your mind and body react.

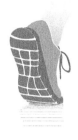

Obstacle Six

Hormonal Imbalances

Hormones 101

Each one of us begins life as a single cell, which continues to divide and differentiate until it culminates in the creation of a completely unique human being. No two women—not even identical twins—are exactly alike. While many of our traits are linked to the genes we inherit, much of the work that goes into crafting our individual differences is carried out by a class of chemicals called hormones.

Various tissues of the body secrete hormones into the bloodstream where they travel to their intended targets—specific cells that know how to read and respond to their chemically encoded instructions. One hormone might tell a cell to grow or stop growing; another, to change its shape or modify its activity. These instructions could make the heart to beat more rapidly or result in hunger signals being sent to the brain.

There are dozens of different hormones acting as chemical messengers inside the female body. Since hormones coordinate or regulate most of our important, physiological processes, their essential actions determine much of what we think and how we feel. They affect everything from our energy, sleep, mood, and motivation to how well we digest our food, respond to stress, recover from an injury, or fight off the flu.

In a very real sense, the quality of a woman's life is largely defined by the status of her hormonal health. When properly balanced, hormones promote optimal female health, performance, and recovery. However, hormonal imbalances are quite common, and they can occur at any age. Because hormones are intricately interrelated and highly interdependent, a shortage (or surplus) of just one can upset the balance of all the others.

 While some hormonal fluctuations are a natural and healthy aspect of a woman's life, those that cause pain or illness are not.

Hormonal imbalances are often caused by a complex set of biochemical interactions that involve more than estrogen and/or progesterone—the two most widely recognized female hormones. While estrogen and progesterone are both critically important to a woman's health, they are small pieces of a much larger puzzle that also includes cortisol, DHEA, thyroid hormone, testosterone, and insulin (among others) that are all managed by the endocrine system.

From a functional perspective, the root cause of a hormonal imbalance can often be traced to lifestyle issues like too much stress or not enough sleep. Environmental variables like noise pollution and toxic chemical exposure are also a large—and growing—problem.

Dietary choices can be a hormonal game changer, too. As we discussed in Chapter One, food provides the body with information. And this information can either help or hinder hormone health. If a woman's diet consists mainly of quick-burning carbohydrates, for example, her blood sugar will fluctuate creating 'peaks and valleys' of energy that will disrupt her endocrine function. Carbohydrate cravings are a common symptom of hormonal dysfunction.

Stress can also influence how well the endocrine system manages and balances a woman's hormones. When released in the proper amount at the appropriate time, adrenaline, epinephrine, and cortisol can all be beneficial; they can improve motivation, concentration, and memory. But too many women are simply too stressed, too often, for too long. Chronic stress will eventually cause the endocrine system to malfunction—in one way or another. And the adrenal glands are frequently the first to be affected.

The Adrenal Glands

The adrenal glands are the two, thumb-sized organs sitting just above the kidneys. Although they aren't very large, they're an integral part of the endocrine system because they manufacture a number of critically important hormones.

The adrenal hormones include the glucocorticoids (primarily cortisol which balances the body's blood sugar and supports a healthy metabolism, stress response, and immune system); the mineralocorticoids (hormones that maintain healthy blood pressure and hydration); the sex hormones (estrogen, progesterone, and testosterone); and adrenaline and epinephrine, acute stress hormones that also affect the body's ability to convert glycogen (stored sugar) into glucose (usable sugar).

The body's response to stress revolves around the release of cortisol. Cortisol's primary function is to help mobilize the body's physiological resources, preparing it for battle—either real or imagined. If you've ever been in a stressful situation and suddenly experienced an immediate and noticeable boost of energy or ability to maintain a razor-sharp focus, that's cortisol at work.

Normally, the adrenal glands release cortisol according to a diurnal or daily rhythm. Cortisol levels are naturally higher in the morning, helping us wake. They decline throughout the day and reach their lowest point in the evening, preparing us for sleep. The predictability of this rhythm, however, can be disrupted by stress.

If the adrenals begin to produce too much cortisol in response to constant stress—physical or mental, real or imagined—their function can become compromised. Blood sugar swings, chronic inflammation, poor joint health, and a weak immune system are just a few of the negative health consequences.

High cortisol levels can also disrupt sleep and lead to unexplained weight gain, particularly around the midsection. This is sometimes referred to as the "famine effect." To the brain, prolonged periods of increased stress signal an impending scarcity or other life-threatening event. As a protective response, the body begins to hoard calories and store them as fat—the safest and slowest-burning form of fuel.

When a woman experiences excessive stress, progesterone is more readily converted to cortisol. And adding extra cortisol to the stress-scarcity equation further activates the female body's adaptive predisposition for converting calories to fat. Once this survival strategy becomes established, the body will habitually allocate more of its resources to protection and preservation; fewer of them will be given to growth, repair, and recovery. This is why it's particularly important for the ill or injured athlete to minimize her level of stress.

Adrenal Fatigue

When stress hormone (cortisol) levels remain chronically elevated, they contribute to the onset of adrenal fatigue—the term used to describe a collective set of symptoms caused by overtaxed adrenal glands. Many women who suffer from adrenal fatigue may look and act relatively normal, and may not have any obvious signs of a physical illness. But they live with varying levels of fatigue and a general sense of unwellness. The need to use coffee or other caffeinated stimulants to get going in the morning and make it through the day is often a tell-tale symptom. The use of stimulants places additional stress on the adrenal glands, perpetuating a destructive cycle.

Adrenal fatigue is a relatively new term that was first used in 1998 by Dr. James L. Wilson, a naturopathic physician. Dr. Wilson's premise was that overstimulation of the adrenal glands by long-term stress could lead to inconsistent levels of cortisol in the bloodstream—at times too much and at others, too little. **In addition to chronic stress, adrenal fatigue can also be caused by:**

- **Eating large amounts of sugar,** which can disrupt the body's hormonal balance and weaken the adrenal glands. During the past 200 years, the average American has gone from eating one pound to more than 50 pounds of sugar a year. Our genes have not had nearly enough time to adapt to this massive increase.
- **Insufficient sleep**. While our ancestors averaged a healthy nine hours of sleep at night, the typical American now sleeps

six. Recent research indicates that women need more sleep than men. Since complete rest is the only time the body can dedicate 100% of its resources to repairing and rebuilding its systems, inadequate sleep will eventually lead to poor adrenal function.
- **Physical trauma.** In some cases, a singular instance of severe, physical trauma can trigger the onset of adrenal fatigue. The most recent research on the subject suggests that traumatic incidents have a deeper and longer-lasting impact on our health than previously thought. A car accident, serious cycling crash, or major surgery are a few examples of events that can trigger adrenal dysfunction.

Adrenal fatigue is quite common, especially among women. Some experts estimate that 60% of all women suffer from some degree of adrenal fatigue. Still, the condition remains unrecognized within the realm of conventional medicine. Unlike other 'official' endocrine disorders (that typically involve some kind of physical damage to the adrenal glands), a medical diagnosis for *hypoadrenia* or low adrenal function currently doesn't exist. Most traditional medical practitioners classify their patients as either having normal adrenal function or complete adrenal failure (known as Addison's disease). There is no 'middle ground' for diagnosis.

Most naturopaths and functional medicine specialists do, however, identify and address the symptoms of adrenal fatigue. And there are a variety of accurate assessment tools available for women to use without a doctor's prescription. Labrix Laboratory (labrix.com) is a great resource for those who are interested in evaluating their adrenal hormone status. Labrix's *Adrenal Hormone Assessment* involves the collection of six saliva samples over the course of a single day which provides for a true, functional evaluation. The resulting six-point graph not only offers a snapshot of the body's daily cortisol curve, but its cortisol awakening response (CAR).

During a normal cortisol awakening response, adrenal hormone levels should increase by 50% the first 30 minutes after waking then begin to progressively drop throughout the afternoon and evening. The significant spike in cortisol is uniquely linked to the stimulus of morning waking. It doesn't happen when we wake from sleep in the middle of the night or finish an afternoon nap. The intensity of the CAR a woman experiences provides some insight into how well her HPA axis (the communication system used by a woman's hypothalamus, pituitary, and adrenal glands) is responding to her total stress load. Women who find it difficult to get out of bed in the morning and do not wake feeling rested and refreshed may have an abnormal cortisol awakening response.

Because a faulty stress response can also affect the body in so many other ways, adrenal fatigue is hard to identify and even harder to study. But its most common symptoms include:

- A systolic (top number) blood pressure reading consistently less than 95
- Dizziness when rising from a lying or seated position
- Difficulty waking in the morning
- Afternoon fatigue
- Insomnia
- Cravings for sugar, salt, or fat
- Frequent illness
- Hormonal imbalances
- Increased PMS and menopausal symptoms
- Acne and other skin problems
- Depression

- Low libido (a lack of interest in sex)
- Poor memory
- Irritability and/or a low stress tolerance

Female athletes with adrenal fatigue can also suffer from poor performance and delayed recovery since their compromised adrenal glands aren't capable of producing enough DHEA (dehydroepiandrosterone). DHEA is the *precursor* or 'parent' hormone that all other strength and recovery hormones are made from.

Adrenal Support

If your adrenal function is compromised, making some dietary and lifestyle adjustments will be necessary. And you may want to consider the use of restorative nutrients including vitamin B5 (pantothenic acid), zinc, essential amino acids, and/or adaptogens such as ashwagandha, holy basil, or bacopa. **Increasing your vitamin C and natural salt intake, however, may be the simplest place to start.**

Vitamin C is critical for proper adrenal function. In fact, the highest concentration of vitamin C housed in the body is found in the adrenal glands, where it's used for hormone production. Since humans can't make their own supply of vitamin C and it's difficult to get enough of it from food, supplementation is often necessary.

Combining vitamin C with certain flavonoids like dihydroquercetin will enhance its absorption and beneficial effects. Since vitamin C can have an osmotic effect in the digestive system, increase your intake slowly (to about 2,000 milligrams a day) in order to prevent diarrhea, nausea, and stomach cramps. I can personally recommend PureSynergy's *Pure Radiance C* as a foundational, food-based formula, and Quicksilver's highly absorbable *Liposomal Vitamin C* for times when you need an additional boost.

The naturally occurring minerals found in unrefined salts are also critical for healthy adrenal function.

Women suffering from adrenal fatigue can benefits from taking an additional eighth to half teaspoon of sea or mineral salt mixed with water the first thing in the morning and once again in the early afternoon. They should also use natural salt to freely season their food. Taste preferences should determine the exact amount of salt consumed. As the adrenal glands become stronger and healthier, the taste of salt will likely become less appealing.

The most convenient way to use salt as a supplement is to make sole (pronounced solay). Sole is water that has been fully saturated with natural salt, transforming it into a mineral-rich brine. Sole should be stored in a glass jar and taken a tablespoon at a time.

How to Make Sole

Sole is water that has been fully saturated with a natural salt. The term *sole* comes from the Latin *sol* meaning sun. To make sole, all you need is a cup of natural salt and a quart-sized mason jar, a Ball wide-mouth, hard plastic lid (available on Amazon), and filtered water. It's absolutely essential to choose a premium-quality brand of unrefined, natural salt for your sole.

Directions:
1. Put 1 cup of salt in a quart-size jar then fill it with filtered water.
2. Close the jar tightly and shake.
3. Allow the mixture to stand overnight.

> If the cup of salt is completely dissolved in the morning, continue to add more salt in small increments until the crystals no longer dissolve. At this point, the water will be completely saturated and ready to use.

Sole has been used as a health remedy for centuries in certain cultures. **In addition to supporting adrenal health, anecdotal and scientific evidence support its ability to:**

- **Improve hydration.** The body naturally repairs and detoxifies during sleep, but it uses a lot of water in the process. This is why we're often thirstier in the morning. The use of sole helps the body rehydrate. It can also restore its electrolyte balance.
- **Support detoxification.** The minerals in sole enhance the body's natural detoxification process. Because it's a natural antibacterial, the use of sole can also help eliminate bad bacteria in the body.
- **Boost energy.** The minerals and stored energy in sole support energy production throughout the day.
- **Improve digestion.** Sole stimulates the digestive system, promoting food absorption and regularity.
- **Control blood sugar.** Studies suggest that sole can reduce and stabilize blood sugar levels.
- **Serve as a natural antihistamine.** This action is likely due to its alkalinizing effects on the body.
- **Prevent muscle cramps.** This action is likely due to its magnesium content.
- **Improve bone health.** Because sole is loaded with alkalinizing minerals, it may play a role in preventing osteoporosis. It may also help to prevent or reduce the severity of varicose veins.
- **Support weight loss.** By improving digestion and nourishing the body at the cellular level, sole can promote weight loss.

- **Boost skin, hair and nail health.** Sole's high mineral content supports healthy skin, hair, and nail growth. It has also been successfully used to fight acne.

Estrogen and Progesterone: A Balancing Act

On a strictly biological level, a woman's body was designed for one very special purpose—reproduction. Because the survival of the species is Mother Nature's number one priority, the protection and preservation of fertility has been hard-wired into the female physiology.

 With its extensive web of connections that affect every system in the body, a woman's hormonal system serves as a sort of physiological internet.

The sheer number and complexity of these connections, however, make it prone to malfunctions and miscommunications. This is particularly true when estrogen and progesterone become imbalanced.

It's a little surprising that estrogen (the collective name for estradiol, estrone, and estriol) and progesterone were discovered less than 100 years ago. At that time, it was thought that these hormones were relevant only to reproduction. Estrogen does regulate the menstrual cycle, and it also controls the development of secondary sex characteristics that prepare the female reproductive system for pregnancy. Progesterone works with estrogen to further prepare the body for the successful implantation of a fertilized egg. If pregnancy does not occur, it initiates the onset of menses.

In addition to these reproductive roles, estrogen and progesterone perform many other vital functions. These hormones influence a woman's body composition as well as her bone and skin health.

And they have powerful effects on the brain and nervous system, too. Since estrogen and progesterone are made from cholesterol, they can easily enter the cell membranes and freely cross the blood/brain barrier. Once inside the central nervous system, the female hormones can alter existing protein and neurotransmitter levels which can significantly affect the brain's structure and function. Forgetfulness, the 'loss of words,' anxiety, depression, and cognitive decline can all be caused by an estrogen/progesterone imbalance.

Estrogen and Estrogen Dominance

When a woman's menstrual cycle is normal, estrogen is the dominant hormone for the first two weeks of the month leading up to ovulation; it's joined and balanced by an increased level of progesterone during the last two. As a woman enters perimenopause and begins to experience anovulatory cycles (when no ovulation occurs), estrogen can often go unopposed, creating an imbalance. Skipping ovulation is, however, only one potential factor contributing to excess estrogen.

Women produce estrogen in their ovaries and they also produce it in their adipose or fat tissues. The more fat cells they have, the more estrogen they make. The more estrogen they make, the more fat they store. It's a vicious cycle that can sometimes spin out of control. Estrogen dominance (having too much estrogen relative to progesterone) is the most common type of female hormone imbalance. Its symptoms include:

- Stubborn weight loss
- Irregular menstrual cycles and/or amenorrhea
- Mood changes, anxiety, and/or depression
- Frequent headaches or migraines

- Insomnia
- Bloating and/or other digestive difficulties
- Thyroid dysfunction
- Reduced sex drive
- Hot flashes
- Fibrocystic breasts
- Unexplained episodes of fatigue
- Uterine fibroids and/or endometriosis

Low progesterone is just one of the many reasons why estrogen becomes dominant. Slow intestinal motility and constipation can also contribute to high estrogen levels. When your elimination is sluggish, unnecessary estrogen isn't moved efficiently through the digestive tract. Given the opportunity to linger in the intestines, it has plenty of opportunity to be reabsorbed and recirculated into the bloodstream. When recycled estrogen is added to what the ovaries and fat cells are already producing, it's easy to see how estrogen levels often become excessive.

Our pervasive exposure to xenoestrogens (foreign estrogens) is another key factor to consider. Xenoestrogens are found in thousands of man-made products. They include the infamous Bisphenol A (BPA) used in the production of soft, pliable plastics (like water bottles). We'll examine xenoestrogens and other hormone disruptors in an upcoming chapter. But here's a short list of those that women are most often exposed to because of their widespread use in conventional health and beauty care products:

- Parabens which are used as a preservative in lotions, haircare products, and cosmetics.
- Phthalates which can be found in plastics and are also used as an emulsifier in skincare creams and topical gels.

- Benzophenones which are frequently found in sunscreens.
- Triclosan which is an antibacterial agent commonly used in deodorants.

Strictly avoid these chemical toxins and any personal care products that contain them. Since the body will absorb a substantial portion of anything that comes in close contact with the skin, cleaning and laundry supplies (that leave a hormone-disrupting residue on clothing) should be carefully selected, too.

As a general rule, it's best to avoid products with the generic term "fragrance" listed on their ingredient labels; it's probably a toxic chemical. If any product has a strong perfume (or chemical) smell, there's a very good chance it's disrupting your hormones. Essential-oil-based fragrances can also smell strong, but they are not hormone disruptors.

 Our exposure to harmful estrogens includes the food we eat.

It's estimated that two-thirds of the cattle raised in the U.S. are given either testosterone or estrogen to expedite their growth. Opting for organic, pasture-raised, and grass-fed meats and full-fat dairy products (which don't contain harmful hormones) can cost a little more. But the health consequences—and associated costs—of consuming unnecessary and unwanted hormones is much greater.

Certain foods also contain natural phytoestrogens (estrogens produced by plants), which are weaker than the endogenous estrogens (those produced inside an organism). When consumed in large amounts, however, phytoestrogens can disrupt the body's hormonal balance. The worst offenders are unfermented soy products and alcohol (especially beer that contains hops).

On the other hand, certain phytoestrogens consumed in small amounts can block the absorption of other harmful estrogens. These beneficial estrogens include the isoflavones found in fermented soy products (such as tempeh, miso, and natto); sunflower and flax seeds. Because they also support bone health, these foods can be especially beneficial for women who are nearing menopause.

Chronic stress can cause estrogen dominance.

The multi-tasking hormone pregnenolone, which is a precursor (parent) to the female sex hormones (estrogen and progesterone) and the stress hormones (adrenaline and cortisol), will go where it's needed most. Under normal circumstances, it provides for making adequate and balanced amounts of both sex and stress hormones. Under duress, however, the body 'steals' the pregnenolone that would otherwise be used for making progesterone to make more cortisol. Since progesterone is what keeps estrogen in check, chronic stress can lead to estrogen dominance.

Stress also affects a woman's ability to ovulate each month. If a woman doesn't ovulate, her body doesn't produce progesterone. Using a bioidentical (identical to what's produced by the body) progesterone supplement can prevent or reverse estrogen dominance. Many women find that oral forms of progesterone have a calming effect. When taken at night, they can make sleeping easier. Others opt for using herbs or natural, over-the-counter progesterone creams to alleviate their symptoms.

While the use of natural progesterone replacements is generally considered safe, it's always a good idea to assess your thyroid, adrenal, estrogen, and progesterone levels before you begin to use any type of supplemental support. I highly recommend the *DUTCH*

(Dried Urine Test for Comprehensive Hormones) *Complete Test* from Precision Analytical. More information on this gold-standard assessment is available at dutchtest.com.

Progesterone Support

While pursuing hormone replacement therapy is always an option, it is possible to improve the female body's ability to produce its own progesterone by nourishing it with foods that are rich in certain nutrients. Although these foods don't contain hormones, their nutrients can help stimulate and support the progesterone production process. **The most beneficial foods include those rich in:**

- **Vitamin C.** Kiwis, oranges, papayas, lemons, strawberries, and tomatoes; bell peppers, broccoli, kale, and Brussels sprouts.
- **Vitamin E.** Sunflower seeds, almonds, hazelnuts, and avocados.
- **Vitamin B6.** Wild-caught salmon, bananas, spinach, and walnuts.
- **Zinc.** Oysters, kefir, spinach, pumpkin seeds, cashews, pasture-raised chicken, wild-caught salmon, grass-fed beef, and mushrooms.
- **Magnesium.** Leafy green vegetables like kale and Swiss chard, cashews, and pumpkin seeds.
- **Fiber,** a nutrient that assists with proper bowel function and, therefore, the elimination of metabolized estrogen. Organic psyllium husks (which are gluten-free); cauliflower, green beans, and berries; flax, hemp, and chia seeds are all good sources of fiber.
- **Sulfur,** a mineral that helps to detoxify the liver by filtering out and eliminating any estrogen metabolites (waste products). Sulfur is found in broccoli, collard greens, kale, Brussels sprouts, and Swiss chard.

- **Natural nitrates and the amino acid L-arginine.** Both support the body's ability to produce nitric oxide—a gas that relaxes the blood vessels for improved circulation and progesterone production. The best food sources of natural nitrates include red beets, arugula, kale, collard greens, spinach, and celery. L-arginine can be found in wild-caught salmon, pasture-raised chicken, pumpkin seeds, walnuts, watermelon, and chickpeas.
- **Dietary cholesterol.** The body requires an adequate amount of cholesterol in order to create pregnenolone, the precursor (parent) of progesterone. Healthy cholesterol can be found in organic egg yolks (from pasture-raised chickens); butter, full-fat yogurt, and cheese (from organic and preferably raw, grass-fed milk); shellfish, sardines, and organ meats.

The Special Situation Called Menopause

Following the onset of menopause, which is marked by the passage of 12 consecutive months with no menstrual period, the female body changes in many ways. Most of these changes are driven by the decreased production of both estrogen and progesterone in the ovaries. Some of these changes can affect sports performance.

Following menopause, a woman's VO2 max gradually decreases which, in turn, reduces her overall capacity for peak athletic performance. Energy production and metabolism also decline, so allowing more recovery time between training sessions will likely become necessary. Exercising in the heat becomes more difficult. The risk of injuries increase as strength and flexibility decrease.

 Over the past two decades, our understanding of estrogen's protective effects of has grown exponentially.

We now know that estrogen plays a significant role in reducing inflammation and stimulating muscular repair; it has even been credited with the ability to prevent delayed onset muscle soreness (DOMS). Estrogen can also ease joint pain during high intensity training by increasing water retention around the joints (which has the added benefit of keeping collagen production high).

Since estrogen is the single, most important factor influencing bone health in women, postmenopausal athletes are at an increased risk for both osteoporosis and stress fractures. Weight-bearing exercise and strength training can improve bone density. Incorporating both of these activities into a regular training regimen becomes even more important as women age.

Postmenopausal women may find that they need to eat differently, too. Lower estrogen levels make carbohydrate utilization more difficult, which creates an increased risk of insulin resistance. For this reason, menopause may be a good time to consider switching to a lower-carbohydrate diet.

Low estrogen and progesterone levels also make older athletes more susceptible to cortisol's negative effects. So postmenopausal women often find it more difficult to manage and adapt to physical, mental, and emotional stress.

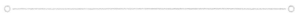

The Dark Side of the Birth Control Pill

For many women, hormonal birth control (the pill) has been a convenient and effective method of preventing pregnancy. It has also been prescribed as a panacea for everything from heavy or missed periods, fatigue, and PMS to cramping, acne, and mood swings. Some women adjust well to the medication, but others suffer from a range of side effects that include nausea, gastrointestinal distress, tender breasts, anxiety, depression, and migraine headaches which all tend to get worse over time.

Although doctors rarely discuss the downsides of the pill, it's important to note that its use upsets the female body's intrinsic, hormonal balance, creating a variety of potential health risks. During a natural menstrual cycle, a woman's estrogen level rises during the first half of the month and falls during the second. The pill disrupts this cycle, keeping estrogen levels consistently high which contributes to estrogen dominance.

High estrogen levels trigger the body's inflammatory response which, in turn, cues the adrenal glands to produce more cortisol in an effort to suppress it (cortisol is anti-inflammatory). Over the long-term, the increased amounts of estrogen and cortisol can impair a woman's adrenal health. In addition, the pill raises levels of a protein called cortisol-binding globulin which holds cortisol hostage, preventing the body from using it. So the excess cortisol being produced can't even be used to address and eliminate the estrogen-induced inflammation it was created to fight.

A number of other hormonal imbalances can also be created.

By utilizing synthetic hormones that change a woman's levels of estrogen and progesterone, the pill can have a negative impact on the thyroid hormones. Women taking birth control pills release more of a substance called thyroid hormone binding globulin (THBG), which essentially holds the 'free' or bioavailable thyroid hormones hostage. They also make more sex hormone binding globulin (SHBG), which captures testosterone; when SHBG levels go up, testosterone levels go down. Although testosterone is widely recognized as a male hormone, women still require an adequate amount of this key, strength and recovery hormone for optimal health, performance, and recovery.

The body is always striving to maintain homeostasis, so it has a variety of feedback systems to prevent chemical imbalances in place. When it receives daily doses of strong, synthetic hormones these feedback systems swing into action. In an effort to prevent a chemical imbalance, the body shuts down its own natural production of estrogen and progesterone. The pill also interferes with a number of other biochemical processes which leave women deficient in hormones like serotonin (which affects her mood) and melatonin (which affects her sleep).

Since the introduction of the pill five decades ago, the effects of synthetic hormones on a woman's emotions, cognition, and memory have remained largely unstudied. But recent research has confirmed that women who use birth control pills for any extended amount of time are more likely to suffer from severe anxiety and clinical depression.

Finally, it appears that birth control pills interfere with digestion and impede nutrient absorption. If you are using (or have used) the pill, be particularly mindful about getting enough magnesium, B vitamins (especially B12 and folic acid), iron, and zinc.

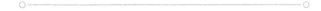

Thyroid Imbalances

According to the American Thyroid Association, roughly 5% of all Americans suffer from *hypothyroidism* (low thyroid function), making it the most prevalent autoimmune disease in North America. Women are at the greatest risk, developing thyroid problems seven times more often than men. One in every eight women will struggle with a thyroid problem at some point during her life.

Located in the neck (about where you'd wear a bowtie), the thyroid gland plays a critical role in cellular metabolism. In fact, the functional integrity of every cell in the body depends on the health of the thyroid gland. The thyroid hormones regulate a range of metabolic processes, including energy production. And they affect the function of the nervous, circulatory, reproductive, and digestive systems.

Under normal circumstances, the pituitary gland releases thyroid-stimulating hormone (TSH), which cues the thyroid gland to produce the thyroid hormone thyroxine (T4). T4 is then converted into tri-iodothyronine (T3), the active or bioavailable thyroid hormone the body can functionally utilize. This conversion process occurs outside the thyroid gland and can be compromised by gastrointestinal issues (like leaky gut syndrome and candida overgrowth), mineral deficiencies (especially zinc and selenium), and interactions with medicines. A thyroid hormone deficiency is created when the body does not produce enough T4 or convert an adequate amount of T3 from T4.

> Sadly, many women needlessly suffer from hypothyroidism because they don't realize that their somewhat random and seemingly unrelated symptoms—fatigue, weight gain, dry or itchy skin, cold intolerance, weak muscles, aching joints, hair loss, depression, poor concentration, heavy or irregular periods, and constipation—are all connected.

While female athletes might appear to be unlikely candidates for hypothyroidism, some are surprised to learn that their lack of strength, energy, endurance, and focus all stem from this often-unrecognized hormonal imbalance.

If comprehensive laboratory test results indicate that your thyroid gland is malfunctioning, you'll need to consult with a medical professional for an appropriate course of treatment. If standard laboratory testing indicates that your thyroid gland is producing an adequate amount of thyroid hormone but you still have symptoms, you may be experiencing what is known as *subclinical hypothyroidism*. In this case, doing some additional assessments may be necessary, but there are a number of supportive strategies you can begin to implement on a sooner-than-later basis.

10 Tips for Managing Poor Thyroid Function

1. **Listen to your body and avoid over training.** In order to achieve their goals, female athletes push themselves both physically and mentally when others would give up. However, pushing the body too hard, too far, and too often can be counterproductive, especially for those with a thyroid imbalance. Training smarter—not harder—and allowing the body a sufficient amount of time to recover between training sessions will build better fitness without compromising thyroid health.

2. **Go gluten free.** A growing body of research suggests that gluten contributes to the onset of thyroid dysfunction. When gluten (a protein found in wheat and other grains) passes through the gut lining and into the bloodstream, the immune system often tags it as a foreign invader and marks it for destruction. At the same time, it often makes another interpretive error—it misidentifies thyroid hormones as gluten, accidentally attacking and eliminating them.

3. **Increase your fiber intake.** Both soluble and insoluble forms of fiber will stimulate the activity of a sluggish digestive tract. When thyroid hormones are low, the entire elimination process slows down. This is why constipation is one of the classic signs of an underactive thyroid gland. Low thyroid function and a lengthy transit time give toxins and other waste products the opportunity to recirculate back into the bloodstream resulting in a range of symptoms that include fatigue, headaches, gas, bloating, acne, and allergies as well as muscle and joint pain.

4. **Limit your intake of raw, cruciferous vegetables.** Broccoli, Brussels sprouts, cabbage, cauliflower, collards, kale are all healthy, nutrient-dense foods. But they contain naturally occurring chemicals called goitrogens (goiter producers) that can interfere with thyroid hormone production. Keep in mind that cooking these vegetables (even by lightly steaming) will inactivate the goitrogens.

5. **Build and maintain a healthy digestive system.** Recent research has shown that intestinal bacteria play a vital role in healthy thyroid function. In fact, intestinal bacteria assist in the conversion of inactive thyroid hormone (T4) to its active form (T3). One of the most important things you can do to promote a healthy and balanced level of 'good' gut bacteria is to eat fermented foods on a regular, daily basis.

6. **Drink warm water with lemon, apple cider vinegar, and honey.** It's a useful tonic for the sluggish digestive system because it encourages intestinal motility, expediting the removal of any toxic waste products that may be accumulating in the gut.

7. **Consider the use of a magnesium supplement** like *MagSRT* from Jigsaw Health. Research indicates that women with hypothyroidism are often magnesium deficient. Adding more

magnesium to your diet can also help the intestinal lining relax, easing constipation.

8. **Include iodine-rich foods in your diet.** Iodine is the main component of both the inactive thyroid hormone T4 (thyroxine) which contains four iodine atoms, and T3 (triiodothyronine), the active form that contains three. Optimal iodine levels are necessary for normal function of both the immune system and thyroid gland as well as the growth and maintenance of healthy breast tissue. Avoid the use of iodized table salt due to its many downsides: it's refined, devoid of beneficial minerals, and often contains harmful additives like aluminum (to prevent caking). Ample sources of naturally occurring iodine can be found in seafood, saltwater fish, sea vegetables (such as kelp), organ meats, turkey breast, black-eyed peas, and dairy products.

9. **Stop drinking fluoridated water.** Fluoride competes with the trace mineral iodine, which is an absolute essential in the production of thyroid hormones. Those who have symptoms of hyperthyroidism (an overactive thyroid), however, should eliminate iodine-rich foods from their diet.

10. **Look for halides and/or toxic chemicals in your urine.** A simple urine assessment can help you to determine how much iodine and how many thyroid-damaging toxins (like bromide, fluoride, and perchlorate) are present in your body. Halides testing is available from Doctor's Data (doctorsdata.com); toxic chemicals from The Great Plains Laboratory (greatplainslaboratory.com).

While it's much less common, hyperthyroidism happens.

An overactive thyroid is sometimes difficult to diagnose because many of its symptoms—nervousness, irritability, increased sweating, a racing heart, hand tremors, anxiety, weight loss, and difficulty sleeping—appear to be stress related. Physical manifestations include a thinning of the skin, brittle hair, hypoglycemic tendencies, and muscular weakness (especially in the upper arms and thighs).

Those suffering from a hyperthyroid condition may have more frequent bowel movements and may lose weight despite a good appetite. Menstrual periods may lighten and/or occur less often. Since hyperthyroidism increases the rate of metabolism, women who suffer from this condition may have a lot of energy upon the initial onset of their imbalance. But over time, as the body begins to break down, fatigue becomes a more common complaint.

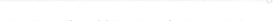

Are Your Thyroid Test Results Accurate?

Unfortunately, routine blood work often fails to detect a significant percentage of thyroid imbalances. In fact, many women who pursue testing are told their lab results are 'normal' and within the standard reference range. Still, they do not feel well. In fact, their symptoms can sometimes be debilitating. Since the thyroid hormones (T4 and T3) are responsible for driving energy production and metabolism at the cellular level, having an adequate amount of thyroid hormone circulating in the bloodstream is essential for optimal physical and mental health.

Symptoms of thyroid insufficiency will vary depending on which systems of a woman's body are most negatively impacted. And the interpretation of these symptoms as a treatable disease will vary based on the specific type of thyroid hormone assessment that's used. Most conventional doctors diagnose thyroid disorders by performing a simple blood test to determine how much TSH (thyroid stimulating hormone) is present in the bloodstream. Some may check levels of total T4, but very few will measure serum levels of free (unbound or bioavailable) T3 and T4 hormones.

Knowing how much unbound or bioavailable T3 and/or T4 the body actually has to work with provides a more accurate assessment of a woman's functional thyroid health. While many women can have relatively normal levels of TSH, their levels of free T3 and/or T4 can still be low. If unbound hormone levels are not assessed, the diagnosis of hypothyroidism will almost certainly be missed.

When TSH levels are found to be abnormally high, it means that the brain has been asking the thyroid gland to work harder; this points to low thyroid function. When TSH values exceed an established test reference range, the symptoms of hypothyroidism are treated with medication. While this seems pretty straightforward, there is some disagreement over how high a woman's TSH level needs to be in order to merit treatment.

Many doctors consider a TSH level above 5ml/U/L a treatable illness. However, the American Association of Clinical Endocrinology recommends treatment for results over 4.1ml/U/L. Meanwhile, the National Academy of Clinical Biochemistry recommends treatment for those reaching just 2.5ml/U/L or more. The variations in recommendations are based on two important considerations—the increased sensitivity of new testing assays that influence the results of more recent research, and flawed reference ranges which have been skewed, over time, to reflect the increasing incidence of thyroid dysfunction (which normalizes higher numbers).

These changes and inconsistencies are important to note because they essentially mean the difference between a sick woman receiving help or being denied treatment. It's equally important to realize that test results falling outside the parameters of an averaged reference range cannot account for unique, biochemical needs of any given individual. While a certain amount of thyroid hormone may be sufficient for one woman, it may be completely inadequate for another; there is simply no such thing as an 'average' woman.

Studies have also shown that thyroid hormone levels can test at normal levels in the blood but be absent in the tissues where they are stored and used. So it appears that there are times when symptoms, not numbers, should weigh more heavily in the decision of who should—or should not—be treated for hypothyroidism

Temperature Matters

While temperature taking is typically associated with checking for a fever, it's a practice that can reveal much about the status of your hormone health. Taking your temperature on a regular and ongoing basis can:

1. Help you identify a thyroid imbalance.
2. Allow you to assess the strength or weakness of your adrenal glands.
3. Give you an objective metric for tracking your hormone health.

The average temperature of a healthy woman with a strong metabolism and normal thyroid function is 98.6 degrees Fahrenheit when measurements are taken daily around 3:00 p.m. If you take your mid-afternoon temperature and find it consistently low, this may mean that your thyroid and/or adrenal glands are underperforming.

The Broda Barnes Assessment Method

Dr. Broda Barnes spent the better part of his medical career addressing undiagnosed thyroid hormone imbalances. He determined that a healthy, waking temperature lies between 97.8 and 98.2 degrees Fahrenheit. A lower temperature points to the possibility of hypothyroidism; a higher temperature to hyperthyroidism.

To implement Dr. Barnes' assessment protocol, take your temperature immediately after you wake up using as little movement as possible. Place a mercury thermometer under your arm and hold it there for 10 minutes. Record the readings for three consecutive days at exactly the same time of day. If you must use a digital thermometer, place it under the tongue and subtract half a degree from each of your readings.

While suboptimal thyroid and adrenal function will both result in low body temperatures, those with poor thyroid function will have consistently low readings; those with poor adrenal function will have readings that fluctuate.

If your goal is to assess or monitor an adrenal fatigue issue, start by determining your daily average temperature (DAT).

This is done by taking your temperature five times throughout the day—before getting out of bed, three times every three hours, and just before bed. To find your DAT, total the five readings and divide the result by five. Date and record your results, repeating this process for five of the next seven days. If a few of your DAT readings differ by more than 0.2 Fahrenheit (higher or lower) from the rest, your adrenal glands may need some support.

Because an increase in progesterone can raise your internal body temperature, it's best to perform temperature tracking prior to day 19 of your menstrual cycle (counting day number one as the day your period began).

While digital thermometers are now the norm, old-fashioned, oral mercury thermometers (available on eBay) are far more accurate. When using a mercury thermometer, it's important to avoid hot or cold beverages for 30 minutes prior to taking your temperature. Be sure to leave the thermometer under your tongue for at least five minutes. If you can't find a mercury thermometer, the next-best alternative is a *Geratherm* (non-mercury) liquid thermometer. While it is not as accurate as a mercury thermometer, it's more reliable than a digital.

Some Additional Assessment Notes

A woman's body temperature will naturally decrease with age. While this is typically a sign of lower cellular energy production and reduced muscle mass metabolism (which are common and expected), it could also be indicative of an age-related thyroid deficiency. Addressing an age-related thyroid insufficiency is imperative as a consistently low body temperature can compromise the function of the immune system.

If you are experiencing higher than normal temperatures without being ill, this can be a sign of low iron, low aldosterone (a steroid hormone that regulates the body's salt/water balance), and/or low estrogen. Your temperature can also increase if you are producing too much adrenaline, which can also surface as heart palpitations and/or anxiety.

The Rhythm of Hormones

Hormones are not static; they are constantly changing, helping the body adapt to myriad internal and external inputs. Our exposure to light and dark is one of the most influential of these. We've known for a long time that the circadian rhythm dictates our ideal sleep and wake schedule. Scientists are now discovering that the entire body runs on a 24-hour clock, a monthly cycle (that's consistent with the phases of the moon); and seasonal and annual cycles, too.

This explains, in part, why night shift workers, long-haul truckers, and those whose sleep-wake schedules are constantly changing have a greater risk of developing certain autoimmune diseases, cancer, cardiovascular disease, obesity, and depression.

Animal and human studies have revealed that the immune system operates according to its own clock which may explain why people have more heart attacks in the morning, or why the aches and pains of arthritis decrease as the day progresses. Learning how to work with the body's internal timing system may one day make it possible to create precisely personalized eating, training, and sleeping schedules for optimal health, performance, and recovery.

Let's take a closer look at what we know about the body's chronological programming.

In a healthy circadian rhythm, a woman's cortisol level will peak first thing in the morning and then drop dramatically around 8.30 a.m. By sundown, it will reach its lowest point. At the same time, her body will begin to release the sleep-inducing hormone melatonin (which is inhibited by light) along with a number of recovery hormones including testosterone, estrogen, and human growth hormone.

Recovery hormones are essential for the repair and replacement of tissues and cells that were damaged or died during the course of the day. If the body doesn't repair and recover well on a consistent basis, it's function will steadily decline over time. Our primitive ancestors had a sleep/wake schedule that was determined by the number of daylight hours they had available. It's fair to assume that they slept more in the winter and less in the summer. Regardless of the season, they slept as much as they could (which was likely somewhere between eight and 12 hours a night).

Things are very different today. Most of us go to bed long after the sun has gone down, some of us not until the wee morning hours of the next day, which may be an expression of our individual chronotype—the behavioral manifestation of the body's biological clock. In general, growth hormone levels tend to peak between 10:00 p.m. and 2:00 a.m. So this is the optimal window of time for physical repair and recovery. Research suggests that our mind mends best between 2:00 and 6:00 a.m. This is why most health experts recommend a minimum of eight hours of sleep each night. The key piece of information to remember is that the timing of the hours you sleep may be just as important as the number.

 We are also learning that when a woman eats may be just as important as what she eats.

A growing body of research suggests that our bodies are most metabolically efficient when our eating patterns are aligned with our circadian rhythms. For the vast majority of us, this means taking our daily meals within an eight to 10 hour window which should open sometime in the morning and close by early evening.

This circadian-based timeframe differs dramatically from that of many American women. In the United States, both men and women eat their meals over a 15-hour (or longer) period. Most days begin with coffee and end with a large dinner followed by a small snack shortly before bed. But these fairly standard eating habits may be disrupting both our circadian rhythms and our metabolic health.

The most recent research conducted by Satchin Panda, author of *The Circadian Code,* suggests that consuming the largest portion of your food earlier in the day is better for health and performance. Dozens of studies demonstrate that the body's ability to regulate blood sugar is better in the morning and afternoon. We burn more calories and digest food more efficiently earlier in the day, too. At night, the lack of sunlight prompts the brain to release (sleep-inducing) melatonin. So eating late in the evening sends conflicting information to the body's internal timing system, interfering with its evening processes by encouraging it to function as if it were still day.

The digestive system also operates according to its own pre-programmed clock, regulating the daily ebb and flow of enzymes, absorption of nutrients, and elimination of waste. The trillions of bacteria that form our intestinal microbiome operate on a daily rhythm as well. In fact, their time schedule is so important that it's actually programmed into our DNA.

While studies suggest that eating earlier in the day is optimal for metabolic health, this doesn't necessarily mean that you should skip dinner. It might, however, make sense to make your breakfast and lunch larger and your evening meal lighter—a practice that many cultures have been implementing for hundreds (if not thousands) of years.

You shouldn't force yourself to eat immediately after you wake up in the morning if you're not hungry, either. In fact, research studies have shown that there are many health and performance benefits to eating during a compressed, eight-hour window of time (between 11:00 a.m. and 7:00 p.m. for example). And that giving your body the opportunity to reach a state of internal autophagy (self-cleaning) by delaying your morning meal can be very beneficial.

 During autophagy, the body's damaged cells and proteins can be recycled into clean-burning energy. Autophagy can encourage the growth of brain, nerve, and heart cells, improve cognitive function, and potentially protect against cancer, neurodegenerative disease, and other illness.

Regardless of when you eat your evening meal, allow at least three hours to pass between dinner and bedtime. This will give your body an opportunity to complete its digestive duties before its internal clock tells it to begin focusing on the extremely important tasks of repair and restoration.

What about exercise? Based on Dr. Panda's circadian research, it appears that morning workout sessions are the best time to focus on longer, slower endurance-based activities; an easy run, spin, or training session built around drill work and technique development is ideal.

Since human performance has been shown to peak in mid to late afternoon, this is the optimal time for strength, power, and higher-intensity interval training. Late afternoon is the ideal time for speed work, heavy weightlifting, and more explosive, plyometric activities; this happens to be the time of day when the majority of all related world records are set.

Assessing your Hormones: Which Test is Best?

Female hormones are complex. Deciding how they are best assessed can be complicated, too.

A woman's hormone levels can change throughout the day, week, month, and year. Most of her hormones are bound to protein, others are active and free. Serum, saliva, and urine assessments all offer a slightly different perspective into the status of a woman's hormone health.

Ideally, all female hormone panels would include a variety of different assessment methods. But even then, the results wouldn't be perfect because hormone levels do fluctuate and lab results will vary. While laboratory assessments offer essential information, they should serve as a guide for understanding the female body's biochemistry instead of a definitive, diagnostic conclusion. Tuning into and trusting how you feel will ultimately offer the most accurate and actionable insights.

Still, it's important to be aware of and informed about the pros and cons of each of the four methods used to assess female hormones.

It's also important to understand that the majority of hormones released into the bloodstream quickly become bound to proteins that essentially inactivate them. In fact, only 1-5% of all the hormones produced by the female body remain unbound and bioavailable. Measuring the levels of these free hormones offers the most useful insights into how much of which ones are functionally affecting the body.

Serum blood tests measure the hormones present in the watery portion of the blood known as the serum. While they are the most common type of assessment used, serum blood testing often offers an incomplete and inaccurate assessment of a woman's functional hormone health because it is primarily used to measure only total hormone levels (which include both the active and inactive forms).

Pros:
- Widely available
- Can be performed along with other serum testing (like a standard blood panel)

Cons:
- Invasive and inconvenient
- Costly without insurance coverage
- Difficult to measure hormones at different times of day, week, or month
- Does not allow for the assessment of free (unbound or bioavailable) estrogen and progesterone

Capillary or dried blood spot assessments use blood from a finger stick (rather than venous blood draw) that is dropped on a specially designed filter card and allowed to dry. Dried blood spot tests were originally developed in the 1960s to screen newborns for phenylketonuria (PKU) with a heel stick, but they have never been widely used despite the distinct advantages they offer over standard serum tests.

Pros:
- Can be performed anywhere
- Blood samples remain stable for weeks
- Can be shipped through the mail
- Inexpensive
- Hormones can be measured multiple times

Cons:
- Many people have an aversion to sticking themselves
- Not all hormones can be tested
- Not widely available; offered only by smaller, specialty labs

Salivary hormone testing has long been used by international researchers who needed a way to measure hormones in remote areas or research settings where blood testing was not practical. In the 1990s, saliva tests were refined and developed for use as at-home test kits for those who wanted a simple, less expensive, and less invasive alternative to serum testing.

Because unbound hormones are small enough to be filtered through the salivary glands, a salivary hormone collection serves as the most meaningful method of assessing hormone health. In addition, the sample collection process is quick and painless. Multiple collections can be taken throughout the course of a day, week, or month allowing for cyclical and/or circadian-based assessments.

Pros:
- Allows for the assessment of all bioavailable hormones
- Painless, convenient, and easy
- Samples remain stable for up to 14 days
- Inexpensive
- Allows for the measurement of hormones at multiple points in time

Cons:
- Allows for the assessment of bioavailable hormones only; additional testing may be needed
- Samples are susceptible to contamination during the collection process
- Not widely available; offered only by smaller, specialty labs

Urinary hormone testing not only measures the excreted levels of all major hormones, but their metabolic by-products (which provides valuable insights into how a woman's body is functionally utilizing the hormones she makes). This extensive information can often uncover imbalances that would otherwise remain unidentified by blood and/or salivary assessments alone.

While urinary testing is commonly used for drug use and pregnancy detection, its application for more extensive hormonal testing is limited as most labs require a 24-hour urine collection period. New and innovative labs like Precision Analytical, however, have simplified the process to include intermittent sample collections taken at specific points of the day.

Pros:
- When paired with saliva, it's the most comprehensive hormone assessment available; the DUTCH test offered by Precision Analytical is the current gold standard
- Collections can be done at home
- Relatively inexpensive

Cons:
- Cannot be used to assess the thyroid hormones
- The collection process can be lengthy (up to 24-hours), inconvenient, and cumbersome

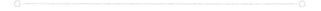

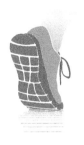

Obstacle Seven

Toxic Overload

Just a few generations ago, most of our material needs could be met through the use of natural resources. Things are very different today. Nearly everything we touch is derived (at least in part) from chemical compounds. In fact, their pervasive presence in our lives has prompted the scientific study of what's commonly known as our *chemical body burden*—the total amount of residue from chemicals that is either stored in or passing through our bodies at any given time.

 According to the Environmental Working Group, women are more predisposed to having a higher chemical body burden than men because they use more 'health' and beauty aids.

In fact, the average American woman uses 12 personal care products containing 168 different chemicals (few of which have been proven safe for human use) every day. And these are just the tip of the toxin iceberg. As a case in point, let's consider the following scenario:

A woman wakes up in the morning on a mattress coated with bromine (a flame-retardant chemical) that emits formaldehyde gas, which her body has been absorbing all night. Walking barefoot toward the bathroom on synthetic carpet, her skin absorbs benzene and styrene, just two of the carcinogenic chemicals used to manufacture it.

Once in the bathroom, she splashes chlorinated tap water on her face. She opens a mouthwash and gargles with a half dozen chemical-based flavors and colors. She picks up her toothpaste, which contains titanium dioxide (a possible carcinogen) and aspartame. After that, she raises her arms to apply a deodorant that contains seven chemicals, including aluminum, parabens (a hormone-disrupting preservative), propylene glycol (a lubricant and suspected cancer agent), phthalates (shown to cause both cancer and infertility), and four additional chemicals disguised as 'fragrance.'

Chances are, she needs to take a few prescription medications which are washed down with water from a plastic bottle and dose of bisphenol A (BPA). By this time, she needs to use the toilet, flushing the remnants of those medications back into the tap water supply for others to unwittingly drink since municipal water suppliers do not test for or filter out medications in the tap water they provide.

Back in the bedroom, she puts on clothes fresh from the dry cleaner that are rife with fumes and residues of trichloroethylene and n-hexane, chemicals known to cause nerve cell damage, memory loss, cardiac abnormalities, and cancer. If her clothing is made of synthetic fibers, she's getting a double dose of plasticizer fumes, breathing them in and absorbing them through her skin.

In the kitchen, she pours herself a bowl of cereal that contains genetically modified corn and soy, high-fructose corn syrup (which contains heavy metals), and a dozen synthetic food additives. Before heading out the door, she grabs her lunch—a sandwich made from pre-packaged meat, that contains nitrates, synthetic hormones, and antibiotics. It's being kept 'fresh' in plastic wrap made with vinyl chloride—one of the deadliest chemicals on earth.

Not yet an hour into her day, she leaves for work where there will be dozens of other toxic chemicals to contend with.

While it's tempting to characterize all chemicals as evil, many were intended to serve a positive purpose. Even dichloro-diphenyl-trichloroethane or DDT, the archvillain of Rachel Carson's 1962 classic book, *Silent Spring,* was once hailed as a "medical miracle" because it killed the mosquitoes that carry both yellow fever and malaria.

It's also tempting to minimize the massive impact toxic chemicals have on our collective wellbeing since many health statistics have actually been improving over the past few decades. These improvements have been documented despite the astonishing number of new chemical compounds being introduced into the environment—and into our bodies—every year.

But the incidence of certain illnesses is increasing.

Since the early 1990s, childhood autism, ADHD, asthma, and allergies have doubled and more than 54% of all American children now suffer from at least one chronic disease. Thirty-eight percent of all American women have at least one chronic health condition, with hypertension, diabetes, and heart disease leading the list. According to the most recent statistics, one in every eight American women will have breast cancer at some point during her life.

Could toxins be playing a role?

Each year, the Environmental Protection Agency reviews an average of 1,700 new chemical compounds. About 90% of them are approved without restrictions (or even a rudimentary review) thanks to the 1976 Toxic Substances Control Act, which requires some proof of a chemical's potential toxicity before it must be tested. In fact, only a quarter of the 84,000 chemicals approved for use in the United States, including the overwhelming majority of those currently used in shampoos, conditioners, deodorants, lotions, perfumes, cosmetics, and other personal care products have ever been tested for toxicity.

 According to the U.S. Centers for Disease Control and the Mount Sinai School of Medicine, the average American woman has hundreds of toxic chemicals in her bloodstream.

Even more disturbing, an astounding 287 toxic chemicals have been detected in umbilical cord blood samples taken from newborns.

Both the International Federation of Gynecology and Obstetrics and the Endocrine Society (the world's oldest and largest organization devoted to hormone research), have expressed concerns that widespread exposure to chemical toxins represents a long-term threat to human reproduction. In the United States, male sperm counts have been falling for decades and are now a full 50% lower than they were 40 years ago. The incidence of infertility and hormone imbalances among women has been rapidly and steadily increasing, too.

Inside the female body, every cell has a hormone receptor site that works like a lock on a door; hormones act like a key. Chemical molecules that are the right shape and size can fit into the lock-like receptor, opening doors they should not be able to open and interfering with normal cellular function. As we discussed in Chapter Three, our physical and mental performance can both be compromised by suboptimal cellular health.

We live in a toxic world. There's simply no denying it.

The regular and ongoing exposure to chemicals, pollutants, and other endocrine-disrupting toxins is an unavoidable aspect of modern life. While it may be impossible to completely eliminate our exposure to all the chemical compounds we come in contact with, we can make choices that will reduce our exposure to many of them. It's a process that may require changing a few habits, like giving up bottled water. And shifting some priorities, like deciding against that Botox® injection or paying more for local, organic produce at the grocery store.

 If the local, organic produce you eat is grown in California, however, it may still be contaminated with toxins.

According to a recent newsletter published by Doctor's Data, "Current irrigation practices permit the use of fracking wastewater for the irrigation of crops such as vegetables and fruits. An Environmental Working Group report found that 95,000 acres (or about a third of all California farmland) is being irrigated with fracking wastewater. Analyses of surface stream water near a fracking site indicated significant thallium contamination."

Thallium is one of the most neurotoxic metals on the planet—more toxic than lead, mercury, cadmium, and arsenic. But since it's less common, it doesn't receive as much attention. The symptoms of thallium toxicity are also random and non-specific, which make them difficult to recognize:

- Fatigue
- Headaches
- Hair loss
- Visual difficulties
- Insomnia
- Depression
- Loss of appetite and weight
- Poor digestion and gastrointestinal distress

It appears that the most significant exposure to thallium comes from vegetables in the Brassica and Spinacia families which include kale, spinach, and lettuce. In California (and possibly elsewhere), produce growers are irrigating their crops with toxic, contaminated water—a practice that's perfectly legal under current U.S. health and safety laws.

There are rumors circulating that the oil and gas companies involved in fracking have intentionally targeted drought-stricken farmers, creating both a market for their *fracking brine* and a regulatory loophole that not only allows them to avoid paying for the proper disposal of their toxic waste water, but to profit from it.

While this matter is currently under further investigation, it may be wise to avoid eating any dark green, leafy vegetables (conventional or organic) grown in the state of California whenever possible.

Zeroing in on Xenoestrogens

Xenoestrogens (false estrogens) are a subset of toxins that merit special attention because they are particularly harmful to women. Whether they are derived from a synthetic or a natural source, xenoestrogens act like real (biological) estrogen in the body, disrupting female hormone balance. Specifically, they promote estrogen dominance, interfere with thyroid hormone production, and inhibit the effects of testosterone, which women need (in small amounts) for healthy bones, brain function, muscular development, metabolism, and energy production.

Natural xenoestrogens include plant-derived phytoestrogens which are sometimes referred to as dietary estrogens because they come from food, primarily unfermented soy products.

Synthetic xenoestrogens include some widely used industrial compounds, such as polychlorinated biphenyls or PCBs (a chlorine compound), bisphenol A or BPA (found in polycarbonate plastics and epoxy resins), and phthalates (which are plasticizers). Take a look at what's kept on the shelves of any grocery store and it's clear to see that much of the food we eat (including natural and organic items) is packaged in polycarbonate plastics made with BPA and phthalates. These synthetic chemicals leach from containers or wrappings into the food and drinks they're holding, especially when heated.

 Recent research has revealed that more than 90% of all brand-name bottled waters are contaminated by xenoestrogens, especially BPA.

BPA is very difficult to avoid because it's found virtually everywhere—in plastic water bottles, soup can liners, all manner of plastic packaging, medical devices, dental sealants—even cash register receipts. A few years ago, after the public became aware of its pervasive (and harmful) presence, many manufacturers removed it from their products and began to advertise them as "BPA-free." Unfortunately, BPA was simply swapped for BPS (Bisphenol S), an equally toxic plastic polymer.

The use of phthalates is even more pervasive.

In addition to being used in all types of packaging, phthalates are found in the coatings of pills and nutritional supplements. They're used as lubricants and binders; and as gelling, emulsifying, and suspending agents. They're found in liquid soaps, laundry detergents, house paints, clothing and upholstery fabrics, nail polishes, and hairsprays.

Despite the creation of the 1997 Packaging and Food Contact Substances Program, safety protections remain lax and ineffective. So it's up to each one of us to take responsibility for assessing and limiting our exposure to harmful food packaging materials.

In theory, any company that manufactures a food container or wrapper must receive approval from the U.S. Food and Drug Administration before it can be used. But there is one sizable and questionable loophole in this rule: substances considered generally recognized as safe (GRAS) are exempt. And the list of GRAS-accepted polymers in packaging is very long.

Plastic manufacturers have been able to deflect the toxicity concerns expressed by the medical and scientific communities due to the successful lobbying efforts of the chemical industry.

According to the Center for Responsive Politics, Dow Chemical spent close to $14 million lobbying both Congress and a number of federal agencies in order to protect their commercial interests in 2016 alone. The American Chemistry Council has spent between five and $13 million on lobbying annually since 2009.

Are Swimming Pools Toxic?

While there are a number of different chemicals used in the treatment of swimming pools, chlorine is the most common because it performs three essential functions: it sanitizes (kills bacteria and germs), oxidizes (controls organic debris from perspiration and body oils), and deters the growth of algae. Unfortunately, there are a variety of health risks associated with its use.

Allergic reactions and skin rashes are common. And although it's relatively rare, chemical burns from abnormally high chlorine levels (typically caused by an equipment malfunction) do occur.

The presence of perchlorates, chemicals that are created as a byproduct of the chlorination process, are also a concern. Perchlorates are structurally similar to a number of other toxins including bromine, fluorine, and radioactive iodine. In commercial applications, they are frequently used in the production of rocket fuel, explosives, fireworks, batteries, bleaches, and fertilizers. While the issue of perchlorate exposure in swimming pools remains under-studied (but appears to be more common in salt-water-based chlorination systems), scientists believe that these hormone-disrupting chemicals are readily absorbed through the oral mucosa (mucous membrane linings) of the mouth. In addition, small amounts of pool water are inadvertently, but regularly, swallowed during any swim.

Chlorine itself can become increasingly toxic when combined with other chemicals, like those found in sunscreens and other personal care products. When mixed, new chemical compounds known as disinfection by-products (DPBs) are created. Chlorine transforms into a chloramine, for example, when it meets ammonia. Sweat and urine both contain ammonia. Chloramines are what cause red, burning, irritated eyes.

When uric acid (another chemical found urine) is mixed with chlorine, cyanogen chloride (CNCl) and trichloramine (NCl3) are both created. CNCl is a toxic compound that can harm the lungs, heart, and central nervous system. NCl3 has been linked to both acute and chronic lung injury. The lungs of swimmers who frequent indoor pools are the most easily compromised by trichloramines. Chronic respiratory ailments (including asthma) are common among elite swimmers. In fact, a 2015 study done by researchers at McMaster University confirmed that approximately 25% of all Olympic-level endurance swimmers suffer from some form of asthma.

Unfortunately, any pool that's used by people will almost certainly contain both sweat and urine. Ernest Blatchley III, a professor of civil engineering at Purdue University, has been studying water quality in pools for more than 20 years. He has found urine in 100% of the pool samples he's tested. In fact, his research shows that the average swimmer deposits about an ounce and a half of urine in the pool during every swim.

Although urine was once thought to be sterile, it's not. And even without urine, a pool would still not be bacteria or virus free. While chlorine kills most germs within minutes, it does not kill them instantly. So when we share a lane with other people, we are sharing their germs, too.

Being exposed to germs isn't necessarily a bad thing since it can help strengthen the immune system.

Avoiding all contact with germs doesn't protect the body from illness, it weakens it. Although you may be able to lessen your chances of getting a particular cold or flu by avoiding public contact, when you inevitably do come down with an illness it may strike with greater force.

Exposure to the bacteria and parasites found in fecal contaminants, however, should absolutely be avoided. Unfortunately, a recent U.S. government study found that nearly 60% of all public pools contained fecal contamination. Fifty-eight percent of the water samples were positive for the bacteria Escherichia coli (E. coli) and the parasites Cryptosporidium (which can live in chlorinated water for up to 10 days) and Giardia (which survive in chlorine for up to two weeks). Most parasitic infections lead to intestinal illness. Certain types of viruses, including the Norovirus, can live for up to 60 minutes in chlorinated water, too.

The World Health Organization states that there are three ways for chemicals to enter the body: they can be inhaled, ingested, or absorbed. When it comes to swimming, all three possibilities exist. The less time you spend in a pool, the lower your risk of developing any symptoms of toxicity will be. If you swim in a chlorinated pool regularly, there are a few things you can do to minimize your chemical exposure:

1. **Swim outdoors whenever possible.** Toxic gases will dissipate when exposed to fresh air.
2. **Reduce your risk of DPB (disinfection by-product) exposure by showering with soap before and after you swim.**

3. **Drink plenty of water after you've been in the pool.** Staying well-hydrated will help flush out any toxic chemical compounds you may have swallowed or absorbed.
4. **If you've been swimming in an indoor pool, make sure to clear your lungs by walking or doing some other form of light, aerobic activity outdoors when you've finished.**

Is Artificial Turf Toxic?

In 1966, the first artificial turf (Monsanto's *Chemgrass*) was installed in the Houston Astrodome, launching the best-known brand name in fake sports fields—*AstroTurf®*. This prominent product placement marked the beginning of the turf era, in which billions of dollars' worth of green plastic replaced much of the real grass grown on American sports fields.

The concept of artificial turf is relatively simple. It's made of three, basic components: plastic blades, the backing material that binds these blades together, and the 'crumb rubber' pellets that are poured in between them, giving the field its cushion and support.

While artificial turf may appear to be a low-maintenance, water-saving, and environmentally friendly alternative to grass, it's very toxic. The product's backing and blades both contain synthetic PFAS chemicals, which are often referred to as "forever chemicals" because they break down slowly and are extremely persistent once they get into the air, soil, water—or the human body.

PFAS is shorthand for *polyfluoroalkyl substances*. These chemicals share a signature bond of fluorine to carbon, which makes them exceptionally durable and long-lasting. PFAS chemicals have been linked to myriad health problems (including cancer), but continue to be widely utilized in a variety of industries due to their ability to repel oil and water. While PFAS chemicals aren't used to make artificial turf, they are used as a lubricant during the manufacturing process (to prevent extruding machines from clogging).

The health risks posed by the PFAS chemicals that end up coating both the blades and backing materials used to create artificial turf fields add to the ongoing concerns about their remaining ingredient—the crumb rubber pellets sprinkled over them.

In 2014, soccer coach Amy Griffin realized that an alarming number of goalkeepers had developed cancer after playing on turf fields. She began to tally all the field sport athletes she could find who had been diagnosed with cancer. By January 2019, her list included 260 young football, baseball, lacrosse, and soccer players.

Because crumb rubber is made from shredded tires, it contains a long list of harmful toxins. The Environmental Protection Agency has confirmed the presence of mercury, lead, arsenic, benzene, and polycyclic aromatic hydrocarbons (a class of chemicals that occur naturally in coal, crude oil, and gasoline) in tires. The non-profit organization Environment and Human Health, Inc. has identified 96 chemicals in the 14 samples of shredded tires it analyzed at Yale University. About half of these chemicals had never been safety tested. Those that had included 11 different carcinogens and 20 assorted compounds known to cause skin, eye, and lung irritation.

Some 40,000 tires, which all contain some combination of dangerous heavy metals, volatile organic compounds (VOCs), and hazardous chemicals are shredded to cover a single artificial turf field. These toxins are absorbed by the skin upon contact. And as the crumb rubber begins to disintegrate over time, microscopic particles break off, become airborne, and are inhaled by athletes. The blades of 'grass' break down, too, forming a toxic, respirable dust that contains significant concentrations of VOCs including benzene, methylene chloride, and a number of polycyclic aromatic hydrocarbons.

Unfortunately, the health risks don't end there. Although artificial turf isn't watered, crabgrass and other weeds can still grow in it. To keep up its finely manicured appearance, groundskeepers apply poisonous weed killers. Fake fields are also routinely treated with toxic biocides to reduce athletes' risk of infections from Methicillin-resistant Staphylococcus aureus or MRSA. MRSA infections can occur from a cut, scrape, or skin abrasion after falling or sliding on artificial turf. The bacteria that cause MRSA infections thrive in the high temperatures artificial turf fields reach—up to 200 degrees Fahrenheit during hot, summer months.

Tennis players take note: the use of synthetic grass to resurface traditional (and much less toxic) hard and clay courts is becoming increasingly popular due to its low cost, easy maintenance, and faster dry time.

Just Say No to GMOs

While they are not really chemicals, GMOs or genetically modified organisms, are potentially toxic food substances—plant, animal, microorganism, or other organism—that have had their DNA altered. The genes from the DNA of one species are essentially extracted and artificially forced into the genes of an unrelated organism. For example, a gene meant to instill frost tolerance in spinach might come from a fish that thrives in icy waters.

The source of foreign genes is unlimited and may come from bacteria, viruses, insects, animals, or even humans. The health effects of the proteins produced by this artificial engineering process remain largely unknown as they have not been adequately or rigorously studied. Genetically modified foods have been linked to toxic and allergic reactions; sick, sterile, and dead livestock; and damage to virtually every organ and system studied in laboratory animals.

 First introduced into the food supply in the mid-1990s, GMOs are now present in almost all processed foods sold in the U.S.

In fact, the number of GMOs available for American commercial use is growing steadily each year. Meanwhile, they have been strictly banned as food ingredients throughout Europe and in many other countries around the world.

The largest genetically modified commercial crops grown in the U.S. include soy, cotton, canola, sugar beets, corn, Hawaiian papaya, zucchini, and yellow squash. GMOs also include any products derived from these sources including soy, canola, and corn oils, soy protein, soy lecithin, cornstarch, corn syrup, and high-fructose corn syrup. Russet potatoes, genetically modified to resist bruising, were introduced in 2015. And genetically engineered, non-browning arctic apples have been deregulated by the U.S. Department of Agriculture and allowed on the market since 2016. The only sure-fire way to avoid genetically modified fruits and vegetables is to buy *certified organic*.

Particular controversy surrounds the use of genetically modified seeds (including soy, corn, canola, cotton, sorghum, and alfalfa) that have an engineered resistance to the highly toxic herbicide glyphosate, which is commonly sold under the commercial name *Roundup*.

The Harmful Effects of Glyphosate

In 1974, the agricultural multinational corporation Monsanto developed a class of agricultural herbicides using glyphosate as the key ingredient. By the 1990s, the company had genetically altered its proprietary corn, soy, and cotton seeds to resist glyphosate herbicides so farmers could use the chemical toxin to kill weeds without killing their crops. Today, Monsanto's *Roundup* is the most widely used weed killer in America. It's also commonly used as a desiccant to dry crops for faster processing. So even non-GMO foods (including wheat, canola, sugar cane, sugar beets, oats, barley, flax, peas, lentils, and other dry beans) are now routinely being sprayed with *Roundup* after they've been harvested.

Glyphosate is literally everywhere. It's in your food and water. It's even in your feminine hygiene products.

Both the state of California and the International Agency for Research on Cancer have done extensive research in cancer epidemiology and have concluded that glyphosate can cause cancer. Yet the Environmental Protection Agency has issued several statements claiming that it is "not likely" to be a human carcinogen. Who should we believe? The IARC is a reputable, world-renowned academic and research institution; the EPA is a political agency. My personal vote stands on the side of objective science.

Cancer-causing properties aside, glyphosate remains a proven endocrine disruptor. And according to the National Institutes of Health, even the smallest dose of an endocrine disruptor can have potentially damaging, long-term effects on reproductive health. Still, *Roundup* is widely used in yards and gardens across America, and farmers routinely spray millions of acres of their *RoundUp*

Ready crops with it each year. Although it's been banned in many countries, its use continues to be virtually unregulated in the U.S.

Glyphosate works by blocking the proteins and minerals essential for plant growth. But the human body mistakenly uses glyphosate in place of the amino acid glycine when it builds proteins, transporting it directly to the muscles and organs. In addition, glyphosate is a major metal chelator; it easily and tightly binds to metals, like aluminum, carrying them directly to the brain.

 Glyphosate makes other chemicals more toxic by blocking certain enzyme pathways in the liver that facilitate the clearing of commonly used compounds, like those found in over-the-counter medications.

These blocked pathways also keep the liver from converting vitamin D3 to its bioavailable or active form, which creates a deficiency. In the intestinal tract, glyphosate kills lactobacillus (a beneficial gut bacteria), which disrupts the entire intestinal microbiome. The gut becomes unhealthy when the beneficial microorganisms housed there can no longer make necessary nutrients (like B vitamins) or important neurotransmitters (like serotonin). When healthy bacteria populations grow weak, harmful pathogens have the chance to multiply and cause chronic inflammation. Chronic inflammation increases the risk of injury and contributes to the onset of almost every known illness.

The extensive list of negative health effects associated with glyphosate exposure includes attention deficient hyperactive disorder (ADHD), Alzheimer's disease, birth defects, autism, heavy metal toxicity, cancer (especially brain, breast, lung, non-Hodgkin's lymphoma, and prostate cancers), celiac disease, gluten intolerance, chronic fatigue, chronic kidney disease, colitis, depression, diabetes, heart disease, hypothyroid, infertility, inflammatory bowel disease, liver disease, miscarriage and stillbirth, ALS (Lou Gehrig's disease), multiple sclerosis, Parkinson's disease, respiratory illnesses, low testosterone, gastritis, metabolic endotoxemia, food allergies, and Crohn's Disease (among others).

Golfers take note: the average U.S. course is treated with approximately 50,000 pounds of pesticides a year—four to seven times the amount utilized in non-organic agriculture. In addition to glyphosate, golf courses are routinely sprayed with *2,4-D* (a powerful herbicide formerly used in the production of Agent Orange that has been linked to the development cancers, neurological disorders, and hypertension); and *chlorpyrifos* (an organophosphate insecticide that has been linked to nervous system dysfunction, lower male and female fertility, spontaneous abortion, stillbirth, and developmental birth defects).

After a course is treated, golfers can accumulate pesticide residue on their clothing and skin, which can be absorbed by the body and/or transferred into the home. Research studies indicate that chlorpyrifos are retained by the skin and internal tissues for at least 120 hours. When pesticide particles and/or vapors become airborne (a process known as *pesticide drift*), they can travel well over 500 yards from their initial application site landing on non-target surfaces like the exterior walls, windows, lawns, and gardens of a private residence. Chlorpyrifos are frequently detected in the dust of golf course community homes, which can build up on interior surfaces including ceiling fans, furniture, bedding, and toys and result in chronic, low-dose toxic exposure.

Prescription Medications

While many of the medicines developed in the last century were derived from the naturally occurring compounds found in plants, bacteria, and fungi, the discovery and development of these drugs has slowed and artificial, man-made compounds have become the new norm. Regardless of whether a medication is naturally or synthetically derived, however, drugs are toxins. While the use of certain medications is sometimes at least a short-term necessity, prescription drugs are now the third leading cause of death in the U.S.

 This shocking statistic is a symptom of a medical treatment model that may ultimately be harming those it was designed to help.

Preventive and naturopathic medicine specialists have long argued that the root cause of most illness is some combination of poor nutrition, unhealthy lifestyle choices, and toxic exposure. People don't nourish their bodies with nutrient-rich foods; they move too little (or too much); and they are constantly being exposed to chemicals. So they are getting sick.

Based on current, conventional medical practices, the symptoms of illness and disease are suppressed with prescription medications (chemicals). And if one of those medications causes side effects, another is prescribed to mask them. Of course, prescription medicines do save, improve, or extend millions of lives. But these benefits are always accompanied by a high risk of side effects. The use of any prescription drug should involve a careful risk/benefit analysis.

Drugs work by interfering with normal cell chemistry; most by disrupting the action of enzymes or by interfering with cellular receptor sites.

Medications are meant to move body chemistry in a favorable direction. But given the complexity of human biochemistry, it's impossible to do just one thing to the body. For every potentially positive effect of a given medication, there's an inevitable domino effect of unintended biochemical reactions that can push the body in an unfavorable and unhealthy direction.

In recent years, the toxic effects of drugs have forced a number of them off the market. New warnings are constantly being issued and new studies are constantly showing drugs to be ineffective or harmful. The production and distribution of *Vioxx* (an anti-inflammatory drug), for example, was banned in 2004 after causing more than 140,000 deaths in the U.S. alone.

Many people are aware that prescription medications can have a toxic effect on the body, but they also do something else—they cause nutritional deficiencies.

Some drugs reduce the appetite, creating an energy imbalance. Some reduce the absorption of nutrients from food and supplements. Some speed metabolism, causing nutrients to be used faster than they can be replaced. Some inhibit enzymes which disrupt the entire metabolic process. Some increase the loss of essential nutrients in the urine (as is the case with diuretics). Those who use multiple medications are at the highest risk of suffering from nutrient deficiencies.

Vaccines

In addition to glyphosate (which comes from the tainted animal tissues used to culture laboratory viruses), vaccines contain a laundry list of toxins including thimerosal (a mercury-containing preservative),

Neomycin (an antibiotic), aluminum salts, formaldehyde, monosodium glutamate, plasdone C, cellulose acetate phthalate, acetone, FD&C yellow #6, aluminum lake dye, glutaraldehyde, 2-phenoxyethanol, polysorbate 80, and 2-phenoxyethanol.

While the Centers for Disease Control and the U.S. Food and Drug Administration maintain that the chemical compounds found in vaccines are harmless, both U.S. government vaccine injury statistics and independent health and safety studies (those not funded or conducted by the pharmaceutical industry) contradict this conclusion. The need for additional, unbiased research remains evident.

X-Rays and CT Scans

Chemicals, GMOs, and medications are all common toxins. Radiation exposure is another. Every time we get an X-ray, we receive a harmful dose of radiation. And for the most part, we're okay with that. We know that a small dose of radiation may not be ideal, but it usually ends up on the winning side of the risk/benefit equation involved in finding out whether that bone in your leg is really broken—or not.

 While X-rays have been used for almost 120 years, the introduction of computed tomography or CT scans in the 1970s was revolutionary and changed the practice of medicine.

CT scans, which use multiple X-ray images, allow doctors to precisely see the inner workings of the human body. After the inventors of the device won the Nobel Prize in 1979, the use of CT scans grew quickly from fewer than three million a year in 1980 to more than 80 million in 2019.

But recent research shows that about one-third of these scans serve little (if any) medical or diagnostic purpose. Even when CT scans are medically necessary, they result in incidental radioactive exposure that can add up to a significant health risk. Researchers estimate that at least 2% of all future cancers in the U.S. (approximately 29,000 cases and 15,000 deaths per year) will result from the overuse of computed tomography.

No one should avoid a necessary CT scan or other imaging test since the risk posed by any single study is relatively small. But remember: the effects of radiation are cumulative. The more you're exposed, the greater your long-term risk of developing some form of cancer will be. Always ask your doctor why he or she is ordering an imaging test and whether your problem could potentially be diagnosed or managed without it.

Those who are interested in calculating the amount of radiation and corresponding risk associated with X-Rays, CT scans, and other diagnostic studies can download the free app made available at xrayrisk.com.

Air Travel

Air travel is another common source of radioactive exposure. And thanks to the introduction of full-body scanners, we're being exposed to a little more before we even board a plane. While many travelers have ongoing concerns about the increased levels of radiation from security procedures, that amount is somewhat trivial. The major source of radiation exposure comes from the flight itself. The higher the altitude, the thinner the air, and the lower our protection from radioactivity (thin air contains fewer radiation-deflecting molecules). Exactly how much radiation are we being exposed to?

A cross-country flight from Boston to Los Angeles is roughly equivalent to a chest X-ray.

The quality of cabin air breathed by passengers, pilots, and crew, however, may present an even more pressing problem.

According to new research from the World Health Organization, toxic cabin air is being linked to everything from cancer to chronic fatigue. Even if the skies are clear at 30,000 feet, the air circulating inside an airplane cabin is not. Most of us know that the recycled and recirculated air we breathe on airplanes isn't perfectly clean. But more recent concerns extend beyond the threat of being exposed to an airborne cold or flu virus.

Nearly all aircraft draw in air, known as bleed air, by way of the plane's compressor. Since the air at high altitudes would otherwise be too thin to meet our oxygen needs, it becomes necessary to use bleed air (along with filtered, recirculated air) to properly pressurize the cabin. It's not unusual, however, for a small amount of oil or hydraulic fluid to leak from the engine into the air, contaminating what the passengers, pilots, and crew members breathe. *Aerotoxic syndrome* is the name given to the increasingly common health complaints suffered by those who are frequently exposed to contaminated cabin air, which is said to smell like dirty socks or a wet dog.

While the possibility of poor air quality isn't exactly cause to cancel your next flight, consider traveling with a facemask (the *N95* variety is best). In addition to reducing your exposure to bacteria, viruses, and bleed air, you'll reduce your exposure to any other airborne toxins inside the plane. Strict fire safety standards require almost every surface on the interior of an airplane to be constructed or coated with flame-retardant chemicals like tris-dichloro-isopropyl-phosphate (TDCPP), which outgas during flights.

Electromagnetic Fields and WiFi Exposure

Electromagnetic fields (EMFs) are invisible, radioactive fields created by electricity that can interact with the energy present in our bodies and in the physical objects around us.

The EMF spectrum includes radio waves, microwaves, infrared, visible light, ultraviolet, X-rays, and gamma rays. Each of these categories is defined by its specific wavelength and frequency. Medical researchers are concerned about the health risks associated with the widespread use of technologies that emit EMFs found on the lower end of the electromagnetic spectrum.

Excessive exposure to radio frequency (RF-EMF) and extremely low frequency (ELF-EMF) radiation is a large and growing concern.

The electricity flowing through the human body plays a vital role in supporting essential functions like growth, metabolism, movement, and thought. Exposure to electromagnetic fields can disrupt this flow of energy, compromising the activities of every organ system and those of the brain. Research suggests that chronic, long-term exposure to EMFs can cause hyperactivity, insomnia, depression, and a shortened attention span.

In addition, the International Agency for Research on Cancer has classified radio frequency (RF) emissions as a possible human carcinogen of the group 2B (a category shared by lead and pesticides). Research conducted by the National Toxicology Program has confirmed a clear link between mobile phone usage and the development of cancer in the hearts, brains, and adrenal glands of rats (which share 97.5% of their working DNA with humans).

RF-EMFs are used in communication systems and generated by mobile phones, utility 'smart' meters, TV remotes, and other wireless networks. While exposure guidelines have been established by the Federal Communications Commission, many parents, doctors, and consumers have become increasingly concerned about the possibility of negative, long-term health effects associated with RF-EMF exposure.

Power lines, electrical networks, and various household appliances such as ovens, microwaves, vacuum cleaners, and hair dryers operate using ELF-EMFs. Research indicates that overexposure to ELF-EMFs can potentially damage the nervous system.

EMF Exposure is rapidly and continuously increasing in our technology-driven world. Within a relatively short time, WiFi has become ubiquitous in our homes, offices, schools, public spaces, and transportation systems. It has become an integral part of our lives, providing us with previously unimaginable convenience. But the radiation emitted from WiFi routers appears to be potentially dangerous at close distances. And chronic, long-term exposure heightens the associated health risks.

Cellular towers are also a source of electromagnetic radiation concern. In fact, several studies have shown an increased cancer risk among those who live within a few hundred meters of one. Other common, but less obvious, sources of radiation include computers, baby monitors, and medical devices.

While few of us are likely to discontinue the use of the technology that most of our lives (and livelihoods) benefit from, there are some simple steps we can take to mitigate its adverse effects:

- **Purchase an *EMF meter* and use it to find out which devices in your home emit the highest EMF levels.** If possible, move your bed away from any major electrical boxes or wires that may be hidden in a wall. Make sure the wall of the adjacent room located behind your bed is clear of any strong activity, too.
- **Turn off your WiFi routers and other devices at night**, or when not in use. You can use a programmable electric timer or install a WiFi 'kill switch' so that this can be done more conveniently or even remotely. Minimizing your exposure to electromagnetic activity during sleep will improve the body's ability to repair and recover.
- **Know where your WiFi router is located.** While there is no clearly defined safe distance from a WiFi router, 40 feet is probably ideal; ten feet is the bare minimum. Remember that radiation from WiFi routers can pass through the walls in your home, so keep this in mind as you evaluate the location and placement of your bed. And remember that children are the most vulnerable to the harmful effects of EMF exposure.
- **Turn off the WiFi or turn on the airplane mode functions of your laptop and mobile phone when you use it.** Consider the use of a wired, external keyboard and mouse so you're not directly touching your computer all day.
- **Use the *night shift* mode on your iPhone, *night mode* on your android, and *blue shade* on your Kindle.** They will help reduce your exposure to EMF's in the current era of light.
- **Purchase an *airtube* headset for your computer and/or mobile phone.** Use speaker phone and airplane mode as often as possible.
- **If you have a wireless/smart utility meter, contact your local service provider to opt out.** In California, you can have your meter replaced for a small fee within a week. If there is no opt

out option available in your area, it is possible to purchase a *Smart Meter Guard*.

- **Don't use a DECT or Digital Enhanced Cordless Communication baby monitor.** While all wireless baby monitors emit radiation, the high-intensity digital aspect of DECT technology requires the constant transmission of microwaves.

Is Bluetooth Technology Safe?

In 2015, 247 scientists from 42 countries expressed their concern about the harmful effects of electromagnetic fields emitted from wireless devices in a joint appeal to both the United Nations and World Health Organization. The scientists cautioned that the potential health risks of chronic EMF exposure included cancer, genetic damage, neurological disorders, learning and memory deficits, and reproductive issues, among others.

Then and now, the Food and Drug Administration and Federal Communications Commission maintain that the EMFs generated by mobile phones and other portable, electronic devices are safe. But research studies conducted in both the U.S. and abroad suggest that they cause brain, salivary gland, thyroid, breast, bone, and brain cancers; DNA and sperm damage, miscarriages, and more.

When we use any type of wireless technology, we are exposing ourselves to radiation.

Much of our modern technology including computers, wireless phones, and WiFi networks all depend on and emit a specific type of low-level EMF called radio frequency radiation (RFR). RFR is essentially the same (but less powerful) type of radioactive energy used by microwave ovens. The key variables that differentiate RFR waves from one another are their frequency (how rapidly they oscillate) and their power. Microwave ovens operate at a much higher frequency and with much greater power than mobile phones.

A difference in range is what separates Bluetooth from mobile phone technology. While a mobile phone antenna picks up signals from distant towers and satellites, a Bluetooth headset receives radioactive signals from just a few feet away.

Proponents of Bluetooth technology tend to focus on the fact that its radiation is non-thermal (doesn't generate heat) and non-ionizing (doesn't produce enough energy to remove an electron from an atom). However, there are more than 1,000 studies linking non-ionizing radiation to harmful effects on mammals. And the fact that Bluetooth devices are non-thermal does not negate or reduce the amount of radioactivity they emit.

What exactly is Bluetooth?

It's a wireless technology that allows for rapid transmission of data between electronic devices over short distances using pulses of short-wavelength radio waves. Invented by Ericsson Mobile in 1989, it was initially called "short-link" radio technology. Bluetooth works by continually transmitting data in small packets of information, up to 800 times per second.

The short wavelength and rapid oscillation of Bluetooth frequencies allow them to penetrate and damage living tissues at the cellular level. This destructive characteristic is what inspired the Russian military to weaponize microwave frequencies during the 1950s.

Specific Absorption Rate (SAR) standards, which define the relative amounts of radioactivity the human body absorbs from an electronic device, have been established by the U.S. government to protect the public from overexposure. And while most Bluetooth devices emit less radiation than current SAR standards permit, they are not subject to any safety inspections.

In addition, scientists almost universally agree that SAR standards are far below what is actually safe.

Because the identified health risks associated with radioactive exposure are cumulative and many people are exposed to radiation from far more than just one Bluetooth device throughout the course of a typical day, the need for additional research on the safety of Bluetooth microwave frequencies seems obvious. Unfortunately, they remain largely unstudied. In fact, it's the lack of any formal studies that has allowed health and communications experts to claim that Bluetooth radiation is safe. In 2018, a U.S. government study conducted by the National Toxicology Program definitively determined that high levels of RFR caused cancer in rats. As a reminder, humans and rats share 97.5% of the same working DNA.

The biggest questions we now face are: how do these findings relate to humans and how much RFR exposure is really safe?

Radiationhealthrisks.com is a recommended resource for those who are interested in exploring these questions—and in learning more about the health risks associated with the rampant and relatively unchecked use of Bluetooth and other wireless technologies.

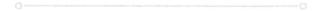

Indoor Air Pollutants

As athletes, we tend to think of air pollution as more of an outdoor concern, but the air in your home or office can also be polluted by formaldehyde (found in furniture and many common wood products including paper bags, waxed paper, and paper towels), trichloroethylene (found in upholstery and other fabrics) and xylene (from caulks, glues, floor polish, pesticides, herbicides, insecticides, and car exhaust). Other common sources of indoor pollutants include mold, pollen, tobacco smoke, radon, and carbon monoxide.

Typically, indoor air quality issues cause temporary discomfort. The symptoms most women experience are relieved as soon as the offending source of pollution is removed. However, some pollutants can cause latent or long-term issues—especially respiratory disease—that take months or years to develop.

 While it's not realistic to think that we can completely control or entirely eliminate all of the environmental toxins we're exposed to, there are some relatively inexpensive, effective, and all-natural solutions that can be used to improve indoor air quality.

Start by filling your house with some air-cleaning plants.

As an outdoor species, English ivy is considered invasive. This fast-growing vine behaves much better indoors by helping to clean the air. According to scientific testing by NASA, it removes xylene, the toxic chemical found in tobacco smoke, car exhaust, and airborne mold.

Anyone with a dust allergy should consider getting a few spider plants. They are exceptionally easy to grow and extremely forgiving of neglect. They can also remove 90% of the toxins in a medium-sized bedroom within a few days. Their leaves are like an all-purpose cleanser absorbing mold, allergens, formaldehyde, and carbon monoxide.

The peace lily is one of the best plants for removing xylene, formaldehyde, and ammonia (commonly found in window cleaners). The thick, leathery rubber plant and the yellow-speckled golden pothos are also powerful formaldehyde purifiers.

If the idea of an air-cleaning plant that thrives on neglect appeals to you, get a snake plant, also called "mother-in-law's tongue." It goes to work at night, absorbing carbon dioxide and releasing oxygen. It also scrubs the air of all the major pollutants including benzene, formaldehyde, trichloroethylene, and xylene.

For even greater protection, consider the installation of a high-quality, whole-house (or individual room) air filter. High-grade HEPA (high-efficiency particulate air) filters from companies such as Austin Air have long been considered the gold-standard.

Mold: the insidious indoor air pollutant.

Molds can live any and everywhere, indoors or out. They propagate by producing spores, which spread through the air. When molds release spores, they also release mycotoxins which make them *toxigenic*. Since mold spores are invisible, they're difficult to avoid. They can find their way into the home through an open window, doorway, or ventilation system; by attaching to objects (like clothing and shoes) or to pets and people. A mold will only flourish, however, if its spores land somewhere that offers the ideal conditions for growth—moisture and a supply of suitable nutrients. Indoor places where mold often appears include areas where water leakages and flooding have occurred; windows where condensation builds up; and spaces where the air doesn't circulate, like inside a cabinet or closet.

Once spores settle and grow, molds can assume a variety of visible forms and textures. They can be white, black, yellow, blue, or green and often look like a discoloration or stain. They can also have a velvety, fuzzy, or rough appearance, depending on the type of mold and where it's growing.

As an indoor air contaminant, black molds (which can range from dark green to gray to black) are a particular concern. These molds thrive in warm, moist environments including bathrooms, kitchens, and basements. They can grow on almost any surface including wood, sheetrock, fabric, cardboard, and paper.

Mycotoxicosis, or mold poisoning, can affect the upper respiratory system with symptoms that are similar to those of a cold or flu. Coughing, wheezing, red or itchy eyes, a stuffy nose and/or itchy skin are other common symptoms. The harmful health effects of airborne mycotoxins can be more severe for those who have pre-existing allergies or asthma and may also include headaches, fatigue, a chronic cough (especially at night), sinusitis, frequent colds, and difficulty breathing. Long-term mold exposure can lead to hair loss, anxiety, confusion or memory loss, numbness in the hands and feet, and unexplained weight gain.

 If you don't see (or smell) mold but still suspect that your home may have an issue, consider hiring a professional mold inspector. They have instruments for mold detection that aren't available to the general public.

Artificial Blue Light

Until the advent of artificial lighting, the sun lit our days and candles, our nights. While previous generations spent their evenings in (relative) darkness, ours are filled with light. While the advent of electrical lighting has allowed us to become infinitely more productive, it does have a downside: a negative impact on our overall health and wellbeing.

Being exposed to blue light can be beneficial during daylight hours because it boosts attention, reaction times, and mood. It is, however, a significant sleep disruptor when used at night. The proliferation of energy-efficient lighting (blue light uses less electricity) and electronics with screens is increasing our exposure to blue light, especially after sundown.

Why is blue light a problem? Because it suppresses the secretion of melatonin, a hormone that plays a key role in initiating and regulating a person's sleep cycle and circadian rhythm. Melatonin production is influenced by the detection of light and dark in the retina of the eye. Any form of light (including dim light) can interfere with circadian rhythms and melatonin secretion. But blue light is particularly problematic.

Harvard researchers conducted an experiment comparing the effects of 6.5 hours of night-time exposure to blue light to that of green light. The blue light suppressed the release of melatonin by the pituitary gland for about twice as long as the green, and it set circadian rhythms back by twice as much (three hours versus an hour and a half). **To protect yourself from blue light at night:**

- **Use warm (red, orange, or yellow toned) lighting as much as possible.** Red light has the least effect on shifting circadian rhythms and suppressing melatonin, although it's not the most practical to work with.
- **Avoid looking at bright screens for at least two to three hours before bed.**
- **If you work a night shift or use a lot of electronic devices in the evening, consider wearing blue-light-blocking glasses** (relatively inexpensive and widely available) or installing an app that filters out blue light wavelengths. *Flux* is a free app (for both PC and Mac) that can be downloaded at justgetflux.

com. Once installed, it will automatically adapt the color of your computer screen to the time of day.
- **Purchase a box set of *TruDark* glasses** that offer different lens shades to block out different light spectrums based on your needs and activities at various times of the day.

Toxins Found in Food

Most of us realize that chemicals, pollution, radiation, pesticides, and medications can all have harmful effects on the body. But it's easy to forget that our total toxic load includes excessive physical and mental stress—and a variety of food-like substances that we may not always recognize as toxins. Artificial sweeteners, food additives, processed grains, hydrogenated vegetable oils, and refined sugars are all prime examples of these.

On a positive note, consumer demand has caused the natural food industry to expand rapidly during the past 10 years. Fresh, organic fruits and vegetables are now commonly available, even in large supermarket chains and big-box retail stores. This is a trend I personally hope will continue. Growing and consuming foods that don't contain harmful chemicals is better for our health, and better for the environment.

While purchasing organic fruits and vegetables is preferable, it's not always possible (or even necessary). Thanks to the annual *Shopper's Guide to Pesticides in Produce* for providing their list of the *Dirty Dozen* and the *Clean Fifteen*. Use these lists as a reference to decide when—or when not to—spend more for organics.

Avoid the Dirty Dozen. Always choose organic when purchasing these most-contaminated fruits and vegetables:

1. Strawberries	5. Grapes	9. Tomatoes
2. Spinach	6. Peaches	10. Celery
3. Nectarines	7. Cherries	11. Potatoes
4. Apples	8. Pears	12. Sweet Bell Peppers

Eat the Clean Fifteen. Because these fruits and vegetables are grown with fewer pesticides, it's less important to buy them organic:

1. Avocados	6. Sweet peas (frozen)	11. Honeydew melons
2. Sweet corn	7. Papayas	12. Kiwis
3. Pineapples	8. Asparagus	13. Cantaloupes
4. Cabbages	9. Mangoes	14. Cauliflower
5. Onions	10. Eggplants	15. Broccoli

The following food-based toxins should also be avoided:

Processed and heated vegetable oils. Especially soy, canola, and corn oils which are all hydrogenated, genetically modified (unless certified organic), and easily damaged by heat. Grapeseed, cottonseed, safflower, sunflower, and peanut oils should also be avoided. Heat-damaged oils promote free radical activity which, in turn, causes chronic inflammation. These are arguably the most harmful food-like substances we can consume. Unfortunately, they are also the most common oils found in commercially fried and restaurant-prepared foods.

Meats and starches cooked at high-temperatures. While grilling and broiling may make meat taste good, these high-heat cooking methods increase the production of harmful chemical compounds known as advanced glycation end products or AGEs inside the body. AGEs increase oxidative stress, feeding chronic inflammation and speeding up the normal process of aging. Their presence in the body is also associated with the onset of many chronic diseases including insulin resistance, type 2 diabetes, cardiovascular disease, rheumatoid arthritis, cataracts, cancer, and kidney disease. Instead of broiling and grilling, opt for a longer, lower-heat cooking method such as steaming, slow, or pressure cooking. Both can be easily accomplished with a time-saving Instant Pot®.

Unfermented soy products contain large amounts of phyto-estrogens, which increase fat production and cause hormonal imbalances in both men and women; enzyme inhibitors, which interfere with protein digestion; and haemagglutinin, which causes red blood cells to clump together hindering oxygen uptake. Because its amino acid structure is imbalanced, the body has a difficult time digesting and utilizing soy. This makes it a poor source of dietary protein.

Fermented soy products like natto, tempeh, and miso, however, are low in the anti-nutrients that prevent the absorption of minerals (like calcium, magnesium, iron, and zinc); they are easier to digest and contain the friendly bacteria (probiotics) that aid digestion and improve nutrient absorption. They are also high in vitamin K2, a nutrient that's essential for strong bones and good cardiovascular health.

Artificial sweeteners including saccharin, acesulfame, aspartame, neotame, and sucralose. Use stevia (an herb) as a non-caloric alternative. Or opt for honey, coconut sugar, maple syrup, or organic, unrefined cane sugar which contain calories but provide the body with beneficial nutrients.

Keep in mind that research done on the use of artificial sweeteners and weight management shows that they have no positive effect.

In fact, they have been linked to an increased risk of weight gain as well as obesity, high blood pressure, diabetes, heart disease, and other chronic health problems.

MSG is an excitotoxin or nerve cell stimulant that has been linked to the onset of a variety of neurological disorders. MSG is commonly used as a flavor enhancer. While it's not an ingredient frequently found on food labels, watch for it disguised as a "natural flavor, spice, or hydrolyzed yeast extract."

Synthetic vitamins, especially antioxidants. Synthetic vitamins are generally not well-recognized or utilized by the body because they are not food. Since they are not easily absorbed, they are not effective and might even be harmful.

Why is the use of antioxidant vitamins a particular concern? Because they are only effective when they work together as a team. Avoid the use of synthetic vitamin A, C, and E supplements as they can create physiological imbalances which, in turn, promote chronic inflammation.

How to Read a PLU Code

Although they may sometimes seem like a nuisance, the stickers or labels attached to fruits and vegetables do more than allow for price scanning at the checkout stand. The price lookup or PLU number printed on the sticker also indicates how a fruit or vegetable was grown. By reading the PLU code, you can tell if a piece of produce is genetically modified, conventionally, or organically grown.

If there are only four numbers ranging from 3000 to 4999 in the PLU, the piece of produce is conventionally grown. PLU codes starting with the number 3 are reserved for irradiated (electronically pasteurized);

6 for pre-cut fruits and vegetables. In codes that contain more digits, the last four indicate produce type. All banana labels, for example, will end in 4011.

If there are five numbers in the PLU code and the first number is an 8, it's a genetically modified fruit or vegetable. Genetically modified produce cannot be classified as organic. Even if it is cultivated without the use of pesticides or other chemicals, it's grown from genetically modified seeds. A genetically engineered (GE) or GMO banana would be labeled 84011.

Keep in mind, however, that not all genetically modified produce may be labeled accordingly. The high volume of new GMO produce being introduced into supermarkets has surpassed the availability of unique code requests that can be processed. Since GMO labeling is currently not mandatory in most states, the more recent GMO fruit and vegetable introductions have simply been assigned a conventional produce code.

If there are five numbers in the PLU code, and the first number is a 9, the produce is organic and non-GMO. An organic banana would be labeled 94011.

When Coffee is Toxic

When consumed in moderation, coffee offers us a variety of health and performance-enhancing benefits. It contains over a thousand bioactive components and is an excellent source of antioxidants. Coffee consumption has been shown to improve exercise performance, fight depression, and boost cognition. It can serve as a potent anti-inflammatory and antifungal agent. Research confirms that it can provide us with some degree of protection against cancer and some studies suggest that it might even help us live longer.

There are a few times when drinking coffee can have adverse effects, but these are typically caused by caffeine (not the coffee itself). Consider switching to decaf if you:

- Have an anxiety or nervous disorder
- Have the CYP1A2 gene (which means you metabolize coffee so slowly that even a cup will leave you feeling anxious or jittery)
- Are pregnant
- Use it to compensate for a chronic lack of sleep

In addition to caffeine, there's another growing concern with coffee—its mycotoxin content. Mycotoxins are formed by molds—tiny fungi that can grow on all kinds of agricultural crops, including coffee, if they're improperly stored. When consumed in large amounts, mycotoxins can be poisonous.

Many different types of mycotoxins exist, but the ones most relevant to coffee crops are the aflatoxin B1 and ochratoxin A. Aflatoxin B1 is a known carcinogen that has particularly harmful effects on the liver. Ochratoxin A has been less studied, but is a possible carcinogen that can harm the brain and kidneys.

While many countries including the entire European Union, South Korea, Singapore, and China regulate the amount of these compounds in their coffee supplies, the U.S. has no safety standards in place. That means many of the substandard beans that are rejected by other countries due to their high mycotoxin content end up being sold and served to Americans.

While the jury is still somewhat out on determining just how harmful mycotoxins are to human health, it's important to remember that they contribute to the body's total toxic load. The heavier the toxic load, the greater the incidence of illness and injury. That little bit of mold in your coffee cup might not seem like such a big deal. But it's important to consider how it may be adding to and/or interacting with the thousands of other chemical and biological toxins you're being exposed to each day.

If you drink coffee on a regular basis, it pays to be picky. As both awareness and demand have increased, there are now a growing number of mycotoxin-free coffees available in the U.S. Some taste better and cost more than others. From a health and performance standpoint, they are all superior to any major brand name.

If you're not willing or able to pay the premium for mold-free beans (such as those from Lifeboost, Natural Force, Peak Performance, and Mindful Coffee), take some time to ferret out the cleanest beans that are available in your budget. For example:

- **Don't shun caffeinated coffee, unless you have a reason to.** Caffeine protects against the growth of molds, which can reduce the number of mycotoxins that end up in your cup.
- **Choose Arabica over Robusta beans.** Even though robusta varieties have higher levels of caffeine, they also contain more mycotoxins.
- **Purchase beans that have been grown in more mountainous regions.** Mold is less apt to grow at higher elevations.
- **Avoid blends.** While they may taste great, there's no way of knowing where the different bean varieties being used have come from. Stick to a single origin product.
- **Look for beans that are shade grown**, a chemical-free method of cultivation that supports (rather than depletes) forest ecosystems.
- **If you drink decaf, make sure the beans you buy have had their caffeine removed through either a water or carbon dioxide process.** Many beans are decaffeinated with chemical solvents including methylene chloride and ethyl acetate.

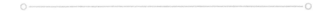

Toxins Found in Personal Care Products

Many women are aware that avoiding processed foods (which contain artificial ingredients and preservatives) can reduce their chemical body burden. Opting out of the use of conventional personal care products is another strategy that can further lighten the load. In fact, what goes on our skin may be even more important than what goes in our mouths. Face and body lotions, creams, cleansers, and cosmetics are just a few of the personal care products that contain ingredients which can be easily absorbed by the body's largest organ.

 While non-toxic, chemical-free alternatives can cost a little more, know that those few extra dollars are going to a good cause—protecting and preserving your health.

While the European Union has banned approximately 1,400 potentially harmful ingredients in the personal care products manufactured there, the U.S. has banned only 30. In fact, the distrust and movement away from American, mass-market brands has prompted many women to experiment with making their own personal care products at home. If you're interested in exercising some of this cost-saving creativity in the kitchen, look online for instructions on how to make everything from cleansers, creams, and cosmetics to shampoos, sunscreens, and scrubs. One excellent resource for recipes is dontmesswithmama.com.

When it comes to purchasing conventional personal care products, pay particular attention to avoiding deodorants and antiperspirants. While they work (deodorants by inhibiting your body's ability to naturally secrete toxins and antiperspirants by clogging your skin follicles to deter sweating), they contain:

- **Aluminum Compounds.** Which clog underarm pores in order to prevent sweating. Aluminum exposure has been strongly linked to Alzheimer's disease and estrogen imbalance.
- **Triclosan or Microban™.** This chemical is used to kill harmful bacteria when it comes in contact with the skin, but it ends up destroying the good along with the bad. While Triclosan has been classified as a pesticide by the U.S. Food and Drug Administration and was banned from use in antibacterial soaps several years ago, it's still found in commercial, name-brand deodorants, shaving creams, and cosmetics. When triclosan is combined with water, it can create chloroform, a carcinogenic gas.
- **Propylene Glycol.** When used on a daily basis, this skin-irritating chemical can cause damage to your central nervous system, heart, and liver.
- **TEA, MEA, and DEA.** Triethanolamine (TEA), monoethanolamine (MEA), and diethanolamine (DEA) are all ethanolamines, ammonia compounds used in cosmetics as emulsifiers or foaming agents. They have been banned as either known or probable carcinogens throughout Europe.

A quick online search will offer a number of DIY recipes for deodorants. Baking soda, lemon juice, essential oils, witch hazel, and coconut oil are just a few of the natural ingredients you can experiment with. There are also a growing number of non-toxic antiperspirants and deodorants now available from companies like Tom's of Maine, Jason, Kopari, Schmidt's, Thinksport, Ursa Major, Earth Mama, and Zion.

 Read labels carefully in order to avoid the use of any creams, lotions, and cosmetics that contain parabens, phthalates, lead (especially common in lipsticks), polyethylene or propylene glycols, or PEGs (petroleum-based compounds that are used to thicken, soften, and gelatinize personal care products), BHT, and BHA.

While finding clean cosmetics can be a challenge, one of the most highly-rated, non-toxic makeup lines is *Origins,* formulated by Dr. Andrew Weil (a well-known integrative medicine specialist). Dr. Weil's products are free of parabens, phthalates, propylene glycol, formaldehyde, sodium lauryl sulfate (SLS) mineral oil, petrolatum, paraffin, diethanolamine (DEA), and polyethylene. Cosmetic and personal care products made by Dr. Hauschka are also toxin-free and widely available. Whole Foods and Vitacost.com offer a wide and easy access to many different brands. But read labels carefully before you buy; not all of their products are 100% non-toxic.

Strictly avoid the use of conventional nail polish and nail polish removers. Less toxic alternatives like those from Orosa, Aila, Sundays, Pacifica, and Zoya are available in retail stores and online. And don't forget to read the labels on all feminine hygiene products, personal lubricants, condoms, and diaphragm gels.

The Dirty Dozen Chemicals

The dirty dozen chemicals are the twelve most commonly identified toxins found in women's cosmetics and personal care products. According to recent research, one in eight of the 82,000 ingredients used in these products are industrial chemicals. Some of these are plasticizers (chemicals that keep concrete soft); others are degreasers (used to get grime off auto parts), and surfactants (which reduce surface tension in products like water-based paints). They include:

1. **BHA and BHT**, which are synthetic antioxidants used as preservatives in lipsticks, moisturizers, and other cosmetics. They are also widely used as food preservatives.

2. **Coal tar dyes,** which are typically listed in the U.S. as "FD&C" or "D&C" followed by a color name and number. P-phenylenediamine is a particularly toxic coal tar dye used in many hair dyes. Darker dyes tend to contain more of it.

3. **Diethanolamine or DEA,** which is used to make personal care products creamy or sudsy. DEA also acts as a pH adjuster, counteracting the acidity of other ingredients. It has been banned in Europe as a known carcinogen.

4. **Dibutyl phthalate or DBP,** which is used mainly in nail products as a solvent for dyes and as a plasticizer that prevents nail polishes from becoming brittle. DBP is also commonly used in polyvinyl chloride plastic (PVC) to make it flexible.

5. **Formaldehyde-releasing agents,** which are typically used as preservatives in cosmetics. They are also used in the production of wood product resins, vinyl flooring, permanent-press fabrics, and toilet bowl cleaners.

6. **Parabens,** which are the most commonly used preservative in the personal care industry. They are known endocrine disruptors. Parabens can be identified by their suffixes which include ethyl, butyl, methyl, and propyl.

7. **Parfum** or "fragrance," which is usually a complex mixture of dozens of chemicals. Some 3,000 chemicals (some more toxic than others) are used as fragrances.

8. **PEG compounds,** which are petroleum-based additives widely used in cosmetics as thickening agents or cream bases. They are also used in a variety of pharmaceutical products including laxatives.

9. **Petrolatum or petroleum jelly,** which is used in creams and lotions to create a barrier that locks moisture in the skin. When added to hair care products, it leaves behind a shiny residue.

10. **Siloxanes,** which are endocrine-disrupting, silicone-based compounds used to soften and moisten creams, lotions, and cosmetics.

11. **Sodium laureth sulfate** is an inexpensive chemical detergent and foaming agent that has been linked to skin irritation, cancer, neurotoxicity, and endocrine disruption.

12. **Triclosan** is a pesticide that's used as a preservative and anti-bacterial agent in a wide variety of cosmetics and personal care products.

Toxins Found in Household Products

The average American home today contains at least 62 toxic chemicals—more than a well-stocked chemistry lab at the turn of the century.

Here are some recommendations for reducing your exposure to toxins at home:

- **Eliminate the use of #3, #6, and #7 plastics whenever possible.** Opt for the use of stiffer #2 (high-density polyethylene) and more pliable but less-toxic #4 (low-density polyethylene) varieties instead. The type of plastic used can be determined by examining the 'chasing arrows' imprint stamped on the bottom of the container in question.

- **Never heat or microwave food in a plastic container.** If a plastic water container has been heated (even by the sun), don't drink from it.
- **Don't refill disposable plastic water bottles.** With repeated re-use, plastic bottles become even more prone to releasing their toxic chemical compounds.
- **Don't drink or eat from Styrofoam** cups or containers Like all plastics, Styrofoam is a petrochemical. Petrochemical exposure has been definitively linked to the onset of developmental, hematological, renal, and immunological disorders.
- **Use glass containers** whenever possible to store food.
- **Avoid the use of plastic wrap** to cover food for storing or microwaving.
- **Avoid canned foods** (especially those that are acidic like tomatoes and pineapple) that do not have a BPA-free lining.
- **Discontinue the use of Teflon™ or other non-stick cookware.** Use ceramic, stainless steel, or cast iron instead.
- **Choose unscented, unbleached, and chlorine-free paper products**, especially tampons, menstrual pads, toilet paper, paper towels, and coffee filters.
- **Use a chlorine filter on your shower heads and a premium, under-sink water filter** on the tap you use for drinking water. Look for a model that allows for the removal of fluoride.
- **Use natural cleaning products** or their old-fashioned predecessors—plain, unscented soap; lemon juice, baking soda, *Borax®*, and vinegar.
- **Discontinue your use of conventional laundry detergents and fabric softeners.** Opt for non-toxic brands like Seventh Generation, Better Life, or Biokleen instead.
- **Pay particular attention to any items that are in constant and direct contact with the skin.** Wash new clothing, bedding,

and towels at least twice before use. Non-organic cotton is particularly toxic.
- **Look for a dry cleaner that uses an advanced wet cleaning or CO2 drying process.** Conventional dry cleaning involves the use of the neurotoxic chemicals perchloroethylene and/or siloxane, which are extremely harmful.
- **Avoid the use of toxic yard and garden products.** Fertilizers and pesticides may keep things green and weed-free, but most aren't good for you—or the environment. The nitrogen runoff from these products harms waterways causing oxygen-depleting algae growth.
- **Make sure to store all gasoline and petroleum-based products in a well-ventilated area** away from any living space. Minimize the amount of time you spend running the engine of your car inside the garage, especially if it's attached to your house.
- **Discontinue the use of any toxic petcare products.** They are harmful to both you and your furry friends. Opt for natural tick and flea shampoos, collars, and related items whenever possible.
- **Stop using conventional air fresheners, perfumes, or any product that contains synthetic fragrances.** Choose those scented with essential oils instead.
- **Try to minimize your use of and exposure to VOCs or volatile organic compounds.** The most common sources of VOCs in the home include paints, varnishes, caulks, and adhesives; vinyl shower curtains; carpeting and vinyl flooring; upholstery and foam insulation; and composite wood products. Fortunately, many low or no-VOC alternatives are now available but are usually more expensive and sometimes require special ordering.

Is Fluoridated Water Safe?

Water fluoridation for the prevention of tooth decay has remained a topic of concern and controversy since it was first used in Michigan in 1945. Those opposed to the now-nationwide process have argued that the chemical may present a wide range of health risks that most notably include damage to the endocrine and nervous systems. A number of recent studies support these (and other) concerns. Two studies conducted in 2015, for example, have linked fluoridation to the increased incidence of ADHD and hypothyroidism. Others argue against water fluoridation on ethical grounds, saying the process forces people to consume a substance they may not know is there—and may not even work.

The efficacy of fluoridated water as a cavity preventer has, in fact, not been proven beyond a shadow of a doubt. While the use of fluoridated toothpastes, which contain synthetic sodium fluoride (NaF), have been well studied and shown to be safe and effective, the use of fluoridated water may offer no oral health benefits at all. As it turns out, drinking fluoride to prevent tooth decay is a lot like drinking sunscreen to prevent sunburn.

While finding fluoridated water in Europe is rare, a full 75% of all U.S. drinking water is currently being treated. Beyond the realms of ethics and efficacy, the health concerns related to this routine practice revolve more around the issue of transparency. Truth be told, 90% of the drinking water in the U.S. isn't being treated with the sodium fluoride found in toothpaste. It's being treated with hydrofluorosilicic acid or HFS, a member of the silicoflouride family. Silicoflourides are an industrial waste product, sold to small towns and large cities by the aluminum manufacturing industry.

So is flouride safe?

It's a question that merits more attention than it can be given here. While the use of floudiated dental care products apperas safe, there are some some valid concerns being expressed about the safety of fluoridated water. In addition to health concerns, there is an ethical issue to consider: does water fluoridation constitute a mass violation of the public's right to make an informed choice for—or against—drinking a toxin that doesn't offer any definitively proven health benefits?

Based on the available evidence, it may be wise to consider the purchase of a high-quality water filter and simply opting out.

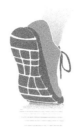

Obstacle Eight

The Lack of Objective Feedback and Guidance

Thanks to the internet and social media, we have more health and fitness advice available than ever before. Some of this information is sound; it's based on objective science. Other information is not as useful because it's based purely on someone's subjective experience or personal opinion.

Even if we could filter out fact from feeling, the sheer volume of information that's available can be overwhelming. There are so many different recommendations that it's often difficult to decide on a singular course of action for improving our health, performance, and recovery. So we end up doing nothing. In addition, changing how we move or what we eat isn't easy; sticking with existing habits that feel like they're working (at least fairly well) requires a lot less energy and effort.

While there is an inherent value to trusting our intuition, making decisions based exclusively on what we think or how we feel isn't always a sound strategy.

Health and performance declines are often slow and insidious, so we gradually adapt to accepting a lower standard of what feels normal because we can't really remember what it's like to feel good. If there is a 'silver lining' to any injury or illness, it may be the opportunity to closely, critically, and objectively evaluate the status of our overall health.

In the past, we relied almost exclusively on the advice provided by a primary care doctor. But in today's standard health care system, physicians are often forced to limit the length of their appointments, spending less and less time with their patients. Because their focus is limited to the diagnosis and treatment of disease, there's little room for asking questions about ketosis or discussing your general lack of energy, late-afternoon sugar cravings, or poor athletic performance.

While a very strong connection exists between these issues and the lifestyle and dietary choices we make, most conventional medical professionals don't know enough about these variables to provide the kind of guidance and support their patients need. In short, the use of dietary and/or lifestyle choices to measurably improve the body's capacity for peak health and performance doesn't fit into the current medical model.

Doctors Don't Know Everything

And they really shouldn't be expected to. They have been trained to diagnose and treat illness, and most are very good at doing that. But making thoroughly informed recommendations on the type and relative balance of fats, proteins, and carbohydrates you should be eating, figuring out why you keep getting injured for no apparent reason, don't sleep well at night, or can't shed those extra pounds around your midsection lies outside the scope of Western medicine. Discussing any of these concerns with your doctor might result in a standard serum chemistry profile as a general screen to rule out the presence of disease. And while insights from this type of laboratory testing can be helpful, verifying the apparent absence of disease doesn't necessarily confirm the presence of health.

 The U.S. currently spends more on health care than any other country in the world. In fact, it spends more than Japan, Germany, France, China, the United Kingdom, Italy, Canada, Brazil, Spain, and Australia combined.

So it would be logical to assume that Americans are the healthiest people in the world; that we are preventing and curing disease—and doing minimal harm in the process. But that simply isn't the case. **Despite spending nearly 16% of our gross domestic product on health care, Americans receive some of the lowest quality of care resulting in some of the least successful outcomes in the developed world.**

Clearly, our costly fixation on disease management isn't winning us any awards. What could—or should—we be doing differently? Some insights can be gained by taking a side-by-side look at disease management versus health care:

Disease Management:	Health Care:
• Masks symptoms without identifying or addressing their underlying cause.	• Treats symptoms by identifying and addressing their underlying cause.
• Implements treatments that often have side effects and unforeseen complications.	• Implements treatments that have mild or no side effects; unrelated symptoms or complaints often improve spontaneously.
• Strives to direct and control care. Patients are not encouraged to participate in or take responsibility for their own health and healing.	• Strives to empower and encourage the patient to play an active role in their own health and healing.
• Views the body as a collection of separate parts, each of which is in need of its own medical specialist.	• Views the body as an integrated and interdependent whole, and recognizes the importance of these connections to health and disease.
• Utilizes assessments and treatments designed to diagnose disease or prevent death.	• Utilizes assessments and recommends treatment programs designed to promote optimal function and health.
• Maintains a focus on managing only identified symptoms of disease.	• Maintains a focus on preventing disease before it happens.
• Implements an indefinite and ongoing treatment plan, usually by encouraging long-term reliance on prescription medications.	• Implements a treatment plan only until the presenting symptoms are resolved.

Adapted from chriskresser.com

Fortunately, there are a large and growing number of options available to those who want to play a more active role in managing their own health care. In addition to working with a naturopath or integrative physician, you could consider hiring a health coach, taking advantage of direct-to-customer laboratory assessments, and/or capitalizing on the use of wearable tracking technology.

Health Coaches

It can sometimes be hard to ask for help. But getting some individual attention and personal guidance can make all the difference when it comes to getting back in the game.

Athletes are pretty familiar with the idea of working with a coach—and with the positive benefits a good coaching relationship can provide. With the assistance of a coach, it becomes possible to set specific, measurable goals and establish a structured, step-by-step plan for reaching them. The same is true when it comes to working with a health coach, except the end result has less to do with achieving a specific fitness goal and more about getting—and staying—well.

> Ultimately, health coaches act as allies helping their clients become their own advocates by encouraging them to become more knowledgeable, self-aware, and capable of making decisions that support their desire to eat, move, and live well—now and for many years to come.

If there have been some seemingly unsolvable health issues standing between you and your health and performance goals, it might be time to seek some additional support.

Gender and Medicine

Until the late 19th century, women were commonly diagnosed with *hysteria*, a conveniently coined term that identifies emotional instability as the root cause of their complaints, particularly those associated with the female reproductive system. When (primarily male) medical practitioners were presented with female patients they couldn't diagnose, they attributed their symptoms to mental instability caused by a "wandering uterus." This baseless explanation can primarily be attributed to the lack of factual research in the realm of female-specific physiology available at that time.

Surprisingly, the medical mindset of treating women—without a clear understanding of their unique physiological or psychological makeup—remained in place until at least the early 1970s. In fact, a 1972 textbook entitled *Gynecology and Obstetrics: Current Diagnosis and Treatment* suggested that nausea during pregnancy was the result of "resentment and ambivalence towards childbearing."

In the late 1970s, legislation was passed to address and prevent gender-based discrimination in medical research. The goal was to ensure that the sample populations used in studies would include both sexes. While we have come a long way, gender bias in medical research is still a problem today.

Women have more strokes than men, but only 38% of all related animal studies (which are required before clinical trials can be conducted on humans) include females. Thyroid disease is at least five times more prevalent among women, yet only 52% of the animal research done in this field of medical study includes females. The vast majority of all drug trial research uses only male mice and other rodents, despite the marked differences in the way males and females (of any species) absorb and process medications.

A 2010 review of gender bias in animal research in 10 biological fields found that a male bias was present in eight disciplines, most prominently in neuroscience where male studies outnumbered the female by five and a half to one. The primary issue is that gender bias in animal research jeopardizes the reproducibility of results in human studies. This is especially concerning given that women experience higher rates of adverse drug reactions than men.

Newer studies, that include statistically significant samples of women, are beginning to reveal some of the profoundly different, gender-related effects prescription medicines can have. The U.S. Food and Drug Administration, for example, has reduced the female-specific dose of *Ambien* (a common sleeping aid) by half. While *Ambien* and other similar products had been sold for many years, it wasn't until tests that included women were done on a new sleeping aid (called *Intermezzo*) that a gender discrepancy was revealed; it became clear that women metabolize the active ingredient used in most sleeping aids significantly slower than men. Until then, it was simply assumed that men and women would have the same response to the drug and that its recommended dose should be the same.

You Can't Improve What You Don't Measure

Measurement is the first step that leads to understanding, then to control, and eventually to improvement. **If you can measure something, you can understand it. If you can understand it, you can control it. If you can control it, you can improve it.**

Beyond doing the standard serum chemistry profile a doctor orders during an annual exam, most women don't have a measurable system for objectively tracking the ongoing status of their health and wellbeing. Many women take nutritional supplements, but don't have a way of assessing their efficacy, either. They rely on faith, a friend's advice, or a social media post when it comes to deciding how much of what products they should be taking. And they are almost always led astray.

 There is a parallel between the way most people make dietary decisions and the process of driving a car around aimlessly.

The objective is to go somewhere, but there are no directions and no way to determine when—or even if—they have arrived.

Before the advent of walk-in labs, the realm of medical testing was an exclusive club that could only be accessed by licensed healthcare practitioners. In those days you would need to make an appointment with your doctor, ask him or her to order the lab assessments you wanted, and explain why you thought they should be considered a medical necessity. Any tests deemed unnecessary could still be ordered, but for 'preventive' or 'informational' purposes only (which makes them ineligible for insurance reimbursement). Obtaining results would require a second appointment.

Things have changed. As most Americans begin to bear more medical costs on an out-of-pocket basis, they are becoming increasingly engaged in and responsible for managing their own health care. While you may or may not have known, it has been possible for you to order your own laboratory assessments for many years. Both their accessibility and affordability has continued to increase as the 'quantified self' movement has gained momentum. As a result, online and walk-in access to laboratory testing is now available in most states.

The labs you choose (either walk-in or online) will contact you directly with results in a time frame that will vary depending on the specific type of tests you've ordered. Typically, results are available on the lab's secure website or by email. Many online assessment sites offer doctor or other healthcare provider consultations along with the results either for free or at a nominal cost.

There are a number of different reasons why many women decide to pursue their own laboratory testing. Some want to have more frequent tests than their doctors are ordering. Some want additional information which requires the use of more extensive testing than a doctor is willing to do. Others are simply curious; they want to learn more about their own body chemistry so they can understand (then control and improve) it.

> **Sorting through the vast number of health assessments that are now available can be a daunting task. But they can be grouped into three basic categories—global health assessments, individual biomarkers, and deeper diagnostic tests.**

Recommended Global Health Assessments

The Serum Chemistry Artificial Intelligence Analyzer

The standard chemistry panel has been around for decades. It evolved as a way to assess the function of critical metabolic pathways and organ function at a time when laboratory testing capabilities were limited in either scope, process, or cost. Once considered the most comprehensive health screen available, the standard blood panel is becoming less and less relevant due to skewed reference ranges (that are based on average results from an increasingly unhealthy population) and/or to shifting medical opinion.

Total cholesterol, for example, was once considered within normal range until it exceeded 250 mg/dl. When high cholesterol was (incorrectly) identified as the primary cause of cardiovascular disease and became an illness that could be treated with prescription medications, the normal reference range was suddenly lowered to 200 mg/dl creating a massive (and profitable) demand for cholesterol-lowering drugs. The bar on what conventional medicine considers normal or abnormal can change, sometimes for questionable reasons.

Even though research has confirmed the essential importance of several 'new' health markers such as vitamin D3 and magnesium, these have yet to be incorporated into the standard chemistry panel. In fact, more biomarkers are being removed from the panel than added due to their cost and/or limited insurance coverage.

 Keep this in mind: since standard panel reference ranges are based on what is considered normal for a full 95% of the U.S. population, it requires a very significant insufficiency or imbalance before any given assessment marker is considered abnormal or out of range.

This creates a problem because results that are classified as normal (despite being suboptimal), may point to more subtle but significant imbalances a busy doctor may not have the time to investigate further.

Sophisticated programs such as those found at bloodsmart.ai and optimaldx.com process the data from a standard serum chemistry panel using an artificial intelligence algorithm that offers a more accurate—and much more comprehensive—assessment of your functional state of health. Based on the 39 different blood chemistry markers it requests, a blood calculator can confirm the presence of:

- Vitamin and mineral deficiencies
- Hormonal and metabolic imbalances
- Immune dysfunction
- Bacterial, viral, and parasitic infections
- Heavy metal and chemical toxicity

Cellular Nutrient Status

Most serum-based tests for nutrient deficiencies measure the number of metabolites circulating in the bloodstream—which can vary based on what foods you've eaten and supplements you've used in the days or hours before your blood sample is drawn. But a company called Spectracell (www.spectracell.com) uses a more advanced and entirely different process to determine what your body's intracellular requirements for vitamins, minerals, amino acids, and antioxidants actually are. The information obtained from this assessment will allow you to determine your body's cellular need for supplemental nutrients. Restoring your nutrient status can lead to significant health and performance improvements.

Cellular Metabolism

A comprehensive *Organic Acids Test* offers a bird's eye view of how well your body's metabolism is functioning at the cellular level. This urine-based assessment from The Great Plains Laboratory (greatplainslaboratory.com) will allow you to identify any irregularities with metabolism, digestion, detoxification, and/or oxygenation that can be improved with dietary and lifestyle interventions.

Advanced Genetic Assessments

Most people have heard of the popular genetic test, *23andme*. While this DNA assessment does offer some good information, particularly for those interested in exploring their ancestry, the technology used in this particular screen is not always accurate, reproducible, and/or functionally relevant. And there are some concerns surrounding the confidentiality of the data gleaned from test results.

The more advanced genetic tests offered by Self Decode (selfdecode.com) in California and DNA Life (dnalife.healthcare) in Denmark have set a new standard in genetic testing. These next-generation DNA tests can help you accurately determine your body's specific nutrient needs while pinpointing any genetic predispositions that may be interfering with your ability to achieve peak health and performance—all with a single saliva sample. Here's a snapshot of just a few of the many things you can learn:

- How efficient your body is at converting sunlight into vitamin D3
- How well your body is coping with the levels of pollution and stress it's being exposed to
- How beneficial high or low-intensity exercise is for your genetic type
- How the presence of a gene that limits the amount of dopamine your body can produce might be affecting your mental health
- Which healthy fats may not be genetically appropriate for you

Individual Health Assessment Markers

While the human body depends on a variety of key nutrients to function fully and efficiently, those listed below are the most important for women to assess and optimize.

Iron

As a female athlete, it is important to understand the difference between a low iron level and anemia. Low iron levels are a detriment to optimal health and performance. They are considered problematic for any athlete because they negatively affect the body's ability to oxygenate itself properly. Anemia, on the other hand, is a disease. The medical diagnosis of anemia indicates that the body's iron status has become depleted enough to cause an illness with symptoms that often include low blood pressure and a rapid heart rate. However, many performance-related problems can be traced to a low iron level in the absence of anemia.

Most conventional medical professionals don't assess ferritin—the marker indicating how much iron the body is actually storing for its functional use. As with many other minerals, a cursory check of your serum iron level is not an accurate indicator of your body's true tissue stores. Just as you can be very low on gas before the low fuel light goes on, serum levels of minerals like iron will not change until the body's tissue stores are extremely low. By measuring your ferritin level, you'll know exactly how much 'gas' you have in your 'tank' so you won't have to wait for the warning light to go on.

While iron deficiency is a much more common concern, female athletes can have high iron—a condition seen almost exclusively in men, who tend to eat more red meat (and calories in general) than women and do not menstruate. Ingesting too much iron from dietary supplements (many multivitamins contain iron), processed foods (which are iron-enriched), and a genetic predisposition all contribute to excessive iron levels.

At even moderately elevated levels, excessive iron can cause inflammation and free radical damage, both of which dramatically increase the risk of cancer, arthritis, and heart disease. Very high levels of iron can cause liver damage, diabetes, and vascular disease.

RBC Magnesium

Despite the key role magnesium plays in energy production, many coaches and athletes don't have it on their health assessment radars.

Since magnesium is not produced by the body, it needs to be sourced daily from magnesium-rich foods including leafy greens, nuts, and seeds. Magnesium deficiency is quite common as dietary surveys indicate more than 70% of the general population doesn't consume enough of it. Magnesium deficiency is especially common among those who eat lots of processed, packaged foods which are devoid of this vital mineral.

While some doctors might test for *serum* magnesium, a deficiency can only be identified once the body's level is extremely low (just like iron). Evaluating *red blood cell* (RBC) magnesium is a more accurate and useful assessment. When a deficiency exists, the body will attempt to satisfy its need for magnesium by stealing it from the cells. By looking directly at the affected red blood cells, it's much easier to determine whether they do (or don't) contain a healthy amount of magnesium.

Vitamin D3

Optimizing your level of vitamin D3 may be the single, most important thing you can do to support your health, performance, and recovery. Vitamin D3 controls or influences almost every physiological process in the body. It's essential for peak athletic performance because it controls muscular strength and recovery, physical reaction time, balance, and coordination. It supports immunity by stimulating the production of antimicrobial peptides (AMPs) and T-cells (a type of lymphocyte), which protect the body from viruses other foreign pathogens.

Many women—including those who train year-round outdoors—are deficient (less than 50 ng/ml) in vitamin D3. The body needs vitamin D3 in order to win the fight infections and/or recover completely from an illness or injury. A less-than-optimal level of this key, physiological factor can inhibit normal hormone production and, as a result, the body's overall health and performance.

Omega-3 Fatty Acids

Essential fatty acids (EFAs) have many functions in the body. In fact, no cell, tissue, gland, or organ can function normally without them. Optimal EFA levels are critical in reducing inflammation, increasing endurance, speeding recovery, protecting the joints, improving mood and concentration, and promoting deeper sleep.

Our EFA status becomes stronger and healthier when we eat foods that are similar to those eaten by our primitive ancestors: antioxidant-rich fruits and vegetables, meats from grazed, ruminant animals, and fats with a high omega-3 to omega-6 EFA ratio. Due to the increased amount of unhealthy, processed fats in our food supply, most Americans don't consume enough natural omega-3 fats (from fish, grass fed meat, seeds such as hemp and chia; and nuts such as macadamias and walnuts) and too many processed omega-6 fats (from corn, soy, canola, sunflower, and safflower oils). These dietary shortfalls have led to performance-reducing imbalances in the ratio of omega-6 to omega-3 fats.

Recent research suggests that we should strive for a low omega-6/omega-3 ratio (less than 3:1) and a high omega-3 index (greater than 10%) in order to reap the full benefits of essential fatty acid supplementation. While you may hear that taking flax, chia, or krill oil is a good solution, studies prove that the best way to achieve these critical ratios is with the regular use of a pure, high-quality fish oil. You can perform an *Omega-3 Index Assessment* at home with a fingerstick kit from Omegaquant (omegaquant.com) or have your blood drawn at any walk-in laboratory or Quest Diagnostics facility to determine your need for essential fatty acid support.

Nitric Oxide

Nitric oxide (NO) is a critical, cellular signaling molecule that declines with age. It not only supports your body's ability to restore its natural antioxidant capacity, but is essential for regulating a variety of cellular metabolic processes including detoxification, blood flow, and energy production.

As women age, their blood vessels become less flexible and this can contribute to many health-related concerns including fatigue, cardiovascular disease, and delayed or incomplete recovery. You can easily assess your NO status at home with the use of a simple salivary *NO test strip* available on Amazon.com or Berkeleywellness.com.

Bone Health Markers

Bone resorption testing is becoming more widely used as an accurate and inexpensive way to measure bone loss. Many integrative and functional medicine specialists now consider assessments such as the *urine NTX* or the *serum CTX* tests invaluable when evaluating osteoporosis since they can identify excessive bone loss before too much damage has occurred. They also allow for the more regular and frequent assessment of bone health status when compared to DEXA (dual-energy x-ray absorptiometry) bone density scans. This means that bone loss can be identified and addressed much sooner and more cost effectively than ever before.

Deeper Diagnostic Tests

Food Sensitivities

The *Food Inflammation Test (FIT)* available from KBMO Diagnostics (kbmodiagnostics.com) is currently one of the most accurate food sensitivity tests available. It can be used to pinpoint any foods that are either causing or contributing to chronic inflammation and/or suboptimal health. FIT test results are accompanied by a personalized nutrition guide. This assessment requires a fingerstick collection and can easily be performed at home.

Hormonal Health

A dried urine metabolites profile known as the *DUTCH Test* available from Precision Analytics Laboratory (dutchtest.com) is the current gold standard in the realm of hormonal assessments. This assessment is a breakthrough in laboratory testing technology which allows for the most comprehensive hormone assessment available.

The *DUTCH Test* is ideal for assessing any hormonal imbalances that may be reducing your potential for health, performance, and recovery. This assessment is particularly insightful for any woman who wants to explore her adrenal hormone status, which plays a key role in determining her overall physical and mental health. Test results provide an analysis of 35 different hormones including cortisol, estrogen, progesterone, testosterone, and DHEA.

Gastrointestinal Health

Gastrointestinal issues are quite common among women. Fortunately, there are several comprehensive assessment tools available that can pinpoint the underlying cause of their symptoms.

The *GI Effects Comprehensive Stool Profile* available through Genova Labs (gdx.net) or the *GI360* profile from Doctor's Data (doctorsdata.com) can reveal important information about the root cause of many common gastrointestinal complaints such as gas, bloating, indigestion, abdominal pain, diarrhea, and constipation.

We now know that the body's microbiome—the collection of bacteria housed in the intestines—has a profoundly important effect on digestion. There are about 1,000 different species of bacteria living in the human microbiome, and each of them plays a different role in supporting (or undermining) our health. Women who have the largest diversity of bacteria in their microbiome tend to enjoy better digestion and elimination. When populations of microbes are insufficient or become imbalanced, digestive difficulties are inevitable because the body can't absorb or utilize food the way it should. Gas, bloating, cramps, and abdominal pain are common symptoms of gut dysbiosis (microbial imbalance).

While all human beings share more than 99% of the same DNA, tremendous diversity exists among us when it comes to our intestinal microbiomes. Because no two women digest or utilize food in the same way, what's health-enhancing for one may be inflammatory for another. Through the use of artificial intelligence, a company called Viome® (viome.com) can provide detailed recommendations on what specific foods and supplements are ideal for improving the health and function of your unique microbiome. Since the gut microbiome influences how macronutrients are broken down and used, its actions will have a direct impact on blood sugar regulation. Women who struggle with insulin resistance may benefit from the insights Viome® provides.

Toxic Load

Because toxins are so pervasive, it's not a question of if you are carrying a toxic load, but of how heavy your load is. For a small donation, you can perform a quick *Visual Contrast Sensitivity* screen by using the online assessment tool available at vcstest.com. Visual contrast sensitivity testing measures your ability to see details at gradually decreasing contrast levels. This assessment is often used as a nonspecific test of neurological function.

There are a number of different variables that can affect a woman's ability to perceive contrast. These include nutritional deficiencies, excessive alcohol consumption, drug or medication use; exposure to endogenous or exogenous neurotoxins and/or biotoxins including volatile organic compounds (VOCs), venom from animal or insect stings or bites; and/or exposure to certain species of mold and mycotoxins, parasites, heavy metals like mercury and lead, and the pathogens responsible for Lyme disease.

More in-depth assessments for chemical and metal toxicity can be done with the *Urinary Toxicity Panel* from Great Plains Laboratories and the *Urinary Toxic Metal Panel* from Doctor's Data. The assessment for toxic metals involves taking 1,250 to 1,500mg of DMSA (a chelating agent) available at Livingsupplements.com prior to a 6-hour urine collection process.

While there are a number of different detoxification options available, I can personally recommend the True Cellular Detox™ program.

Biological Age

Women age at different rates depending on their genes, diet, training load, lifestyle, stress resilience, and environment. Currently, there are two different tools that can be used to accurately assess your biological age.

TruAge® uses something called an epigenetic clock to measure a process known as DNA methylation (the process that influences gene expression). Numerous studies have shown that dietary and lifestyle choices, physical and emotional stress, and exposure to environmental toxins can alter the DNA methylation patterns in our cells. When DNA is altered, evidence is left in the form of a mark. More marks indicate more advanced aging.

Life Length Labs in Madrid, Spain currently offers the most advanced *Telomere Assessment*. Telomeres are small tags at the end of our DNA strands (similar to the ends of shoelaces) that grow shorter and shorter as we age. As telomeres begin to shorten, the body begins to age. Telomere length is an important biomarker in the body. By assessing it, you can determine both your biological age and cellular health status. Using Life Length's technology, you can develop a personalized plan for slowing your aging process down.

Wearable Tracking Technology

We've come a long way since 1975 when the calculator watch—the world's first modern, wearable technology—was launched and became an overnight sensation. No longer a novelty, wearable technology has become a common aspect of our everyday lives, especially for performance-oriented athletes who rely on it as a training assessment tool.

 With an ever-increasing number of health and fitness tracking apps available, we can gain more objective insights into how our bodies physiologically respond to how we train, eat, and sleep.

Tracking just a few, key variables will allow you to objectively assess your health and fitness gains.

Heart Rate Variability

Heart Rate Variability or HRV has emerged as one of the most useful apps for assessing and tracking your body's general health, performance, and recovery status. Researchers and physiologists have been tracking and utilizing HRV for decades. In general, high heart rate variability indicates strong cardiovascular fitness and good overall health. As a practical application, it tells us how well-recovered and ready to train we are on any given day.

Although it may sound counterintuitive, a healthy heart beat should contain some slight irregularities; it should not function like a clock. Women typically have a higher heart rate variability than men.

Using HRV, it's possible to determine when the body has reached a state of overtraining. With its adaptive resources depleted, the body down regulates its systems causing significant health, performance, and recovery declines. Consistently low HRV readings are associated with chronic inflammation, poor immune response, and an autonomic nervous system imbalance. There is no optimal or goal HRV range to strive for because trends are unique to every individual. However, if a very fit athlete who tends to have an HRV score above 70 suddenly sees it drop below 60, this would be a warning sign that some additional recovery time is required.

Tracking your HRV is easy. All it requires is a Bluetooth-enabled heart rate monitor and an HRV application. While there are a number of different HRV applications available, I recommend the free *Elite HRV* app paired with the Polar *H10* heart rate strap (*Fitbit* and other wrist-based data will not be accurate). A heart rate variability reading takes just three minutes and is best done in the morning upon waking. After tracking your HRV on a daily basis for about two weeks, you'll be able to see how your autonomic nervous system is functioning. At this point, you will also begin to see what normal or typical ranges and patterns are emerging for you. These form the foundation of your measurement parameters or HRV trends. It is essential to track and follow trends as opposed to relying on individual readings, and to be consistent with taking morning readings.

 When used for biofeedback, an athlete can take live readings of her HRV that will provide real-time information about how changes in thinking, emotions, breathing patterns, and other behaviors immediately impact the activity of her autonomic nervous system.

Because HRV can react to changes in the body even faster than our heart rate can reveal, it can provide us with immediate insights into the status of our physical and mental wellbeing. By measuring HRV regularly, it's possible to watch the body shift between sympathetic and parasympathetic dominance. Athletes who have difficulty establishing a healthy balance between their sympathetic and parasympathetic states can use HRV as a biofeedback training tool.

There is clear evidence supporting the benefits of HRV-based biofeedback. It has been shown to improve otherwise unmanageable depression, for example. And it can help an individual increase her body awareness and control. Breathing and meditation practices can cause marked improvements in both HRV and autonomic nervous system balance.

Sleep and Performance Metrics

While measuring your HRV every morning can provide powerful insights into your overall health and fitness status, biotrackers such as the *BioStrap™* and *Oura Ring* take things to a next level by providing for the around-the-clock measurement of stress (both physical and mental) and sleep metrics. If the constant wearing of a wrist strap or ring isn't right for you, consider the purchase of a sleep tracking device like the *Emfit QS* (emfit.com) which works through a pad placed under your mattress.

Other Measurement Tools

Blood Pressure

Both high and low blood pressure are symptoms of a body out of balance. Monitoring your blood pressure on a regular and ongoing basis have practical applications that extend beyond the management and prevention of heart disease. For example, checking your blood pressure each day upon waking can offer specific insights into your body's metabolic and autonomic function. Ideal blood pressure levels can range from 100/60 to 120/80 mmHg.

Women who are recovering from adrenal fatigue should pay particular attention to monitoring their change in blood pressure when they stand. If a woman's systolic blood pressure drops under 95mmHg and/or her diastolic falls more than 10mmHg within two to five minutes after standing, she may be suffering from adrenal fatigue and/or autonomic nervous system dysfunction.

Body Temperature

Taking your temperature is a simple, inexpensive tool for assessing the overall status of your hormonal health.

In general, the average temperature of a female adult with a healthy thyroid gland and strong thyroid metabolism is 98.6 degrees Fahrenheit in the mid-afternoon. If you take your temperature daily at 3:00 p.m. and find that it's consistently lower than 98.6, your thyroid and/or adrenal glands may be underperforming.

Lean Body Mass

In recent years, the use of bioelectrical impedance analysis (BIA) for body composition assessment is a feature that's been added to the standard bathroom scale. Stepping on built-in foot sensors triggers the release of a harmless electrical current which is passed through the lower half of the body. Because muscle contains more water than fat, it offers less resistance and conducts electricity better.

Based on the rate at which the electrical current travels, the scale utilizes a pre-programmed formula to calculate fat-free body mass.

It then uses input data (including height, weight, gender, and age) to determine body fat percentage. Carrying too much—or too little—body fat can negatively affect a female athlete's health, performance, and recovery.

Although they are easy, convenient, and inexpensive, BIA scales are not highly accurate. Studies have found that different body composition scales produce variable readings; and these readings often differ from traditional body composition assessments (like body circumference and skinfold measurements). In addition, scales with only foot electrodes tend to underestimate the amount of body fat in those who carry more and overestimate it in those who carry less.

Despite their inaccuracies, however, using a scale with BIA technology can help you detect any major, body composition changes that may indicate a decline in the status of your health and wellbeing. The use of a BIA scale (like the *Renpho Smart Scale, Withings Body Plus, or Fitbit Aria 2)* at regular weekly or monthly intervals can, for example, allow you to identify trends (like the loss of lean muscle mass) that will allow you to take corrective actions (like placing more emphasis on strength training, increasing your protein intake and/or supplementing with an essential amino acid formula).

In addition to tracking body composition trends, the use of a smart scale makes it possible to maintain an awareness of other key metrics including your hydration status, bone mass, and basal metabolic rate (BMR). Even though the readings may not be 100% accurate, they will be more consistent and insightful if they are always taken first thing in the morning prior to eating or drinking.

Brain Health

Fatigue can have harmful effects on the body's ability to perform and recover. Using the free, online *Reaction Time Test* at Humanbenchmark.com is a quick and convenient tool for monitoring your level of fatigue.

Brain Gauge from Cortical Metrics offers another fun and convenient way to obtain meaningful data that can provide a clear picture of how well you rested and/or recovered you are. It will also provide a platform for monitoring the effects of any nutrition and/or detoxification program you may be following. The program's powerful data analytics is based on eight, essential components of brain health: speed, focus, fatigue, accuracy, sequencing, timing perception, plasticity, and connectivity. The resulting comprehensive mental fitness score offers guidance in making health and performance-enhancing adjustments to your training, lifestyle, and diet.

 While all of these apps and devices can provide you with a lot of information, working with an experienced coach who knows how to practically apply it will multiply your end benefits.

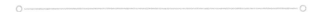

Let's Shake on That: The Importance of Grip Strength

Staying active is one of the most valuable health tools we have. The more we sit, the faster we age. The more we (strategically and appropriately) move, the stronger our metabolism becomes—and the better we look, feel, think, learn, and remember.

Different types and intensities of exercise have different effects on our physiology. This is especially true when it comes to preserving muscle mass and metabolic might as we age. Intense exercise is more effective in preserving our BMR (basal metabolic rate) and preventing muscle loss. Lower-intensity activity also serves an important purpose (especially for those whose health and performance goals include fat loss), but it doesn't do as much to support a strong metabolism.

The definition of high-intensity is, of course, relative. And it can vary greatly from woman to woman, depending on how well an individual's body has adapted to any given form of exercise.

One of the best ways to determine your current state of physiological fitness (it's even better than doing a VO2 max assessment) is to perform a simple hand grip test. The stronger your grip, the slower you're aging. If your grip is strong, chances are that you are strong; you have lots of lean body mass, strong connective tissues, a dense skeleton, and the motor skills necessary to coordinate the combined use of all these things. It's not too difficult to see why strength and resistance training becomes a priority with age.

Regardless of your chosen sport or the level at which you compete, it's important to lift heavy things on a regular, ongoing basis. You don't need to spend hours and hours in the gym. A lot can be accomplished by investing 30 to 45 minutes, once or twice a week.

Is Age a Matter of Mind?

Can forgetting about how old you are make your body younger? Based on scientific research, the answer appears to be "yes."

In 1979, psychologist Ellen Langer and her students refurbished an old monastery in Peterborough, New Hampshire to resemble a place that would have existed two decades earlier. They invited a group of elderly men in their late 70s and early 80s to spend a week there, living as they did in 1959. Her idea was to return the men (at least in their minds) to a time when they were younger in order to assess the physiological consequences.

Every day, Langer and her students met with the men to discuss 'current' events like the first U.S. satellite launch and Fidel Castro entering Havana after his march across Cuba. They talked about newly released books like Ian Fleming's *Goldfinger* and Leon Uris' *Exodus*. They watched Ed Sullivan, Jack Benny, and Jackie Gleason on a black-and-white TV, listened to Nat King Cole on the radio, and saw Marilyn Monroe in *Some Like It Hot*.

When Langer studied the men after a week of sensory and mindful immersion in the past, she found that their memory, vision, hearing, and even physical strength had improved. She compared the traits to those of a control group who had also spent a week in retreat. The control group, however, was told the experiment was simply about reminiscing; they weren't given the opportunity to live as if it were actually 1959.

Langer never published her results. She didn't have the funding to properly control the second group and didn't want to release her data in a second-rate journal. But the experience never left her mind. Years later she conducted a study on patients with type 2 diabetes. Forty-six subjects played computer games for an hour and a half. They had to switch games every 15 minutes. One group had a properly working clock; one had a clock that kept time slowly; the remaining group had a clock that was sped up. Langer wanted to know if her participants' blood sugar levels would follow real or perceived time. Incredibly, perceived time won. How the subjects perceived or thought about time actually influenced their metabolism.

Langer's work shows that when it comes to the process of aging, it's not necessarily the body influencing the mind. Your thoughts and beliefs about aging play an equally important role in determining your mental and physical capacities.

Do you believe your age limits your physical and mental abilities? Do you use your age as an excuse for not trying new things? Do you spend more time thinking about what was instead of planning for what's to come? The answers to these questions reflect your mindset. And as Langer's research shows, the mind can play tricks on the body—in many surprising and beneficial ways.

Conclusion

Clearly, there's no one-size-fits-all solution for maximizing your body's innate capacity for optimal health, performance, and recovery. Making the 'right' lifestyle and dietary choices is a balancing act that leaves ample room for personal experimentation. And there are contradictions to be found almost every time you are faced with a decision—eat nuts as a snack because they are a slow and clean-burning source of fuel or avoid them because they contain phytates which can interfere with the absorption of other nutrients?

Getting back in the game can often be a perplexing process. So what's a girl to do?

Avoid extremes. Who we are is literally a function of what we eat. So it's important to remember that our diets can't exist as an entity set apart from the rest of our lives. Ideally, our food and lifestyle choices should be not only harmonious, but health enhancing. Focus on the 'big picture' and strive to eliminate the inconsistencies that might be interfering with your personal health and performance goals.

Listen to your body. We are all individuals, unique in both personality and physiology. It is often said that when it comes to nutrition, we are all an "n" or research study sample of one. Getting back in the game will likely require some combination of science and intuition. Taking the time to develop and hone your instincts can serve you well. But include at least a few objective assessments in your long-term game plan.

Arm yourself with (trusted) information. And take responsibility for optimizing your own health and wellbeing. While primary care doctors can help manage symptoms and save lives, addressing lifestyle-related concerns lies outside the scope of their practice. Many doctors admit that they don't have much formal training in lifestyle management or nutrition. In fact, surveys show that most graduating medical students rate their nutrition preparation as "inadequate."

Consider working with a health coach. Health coaches offer an invaluable source of support because they can help fill and bridge the gaps that exist in our current health care system. While they are not *Registered Dieticians* (RD's) or *Certified Nutritionists* (CN's), health coaches can act as supportive mentors and wellness authorities who can help their clients reach—or even exceed—their health and performance goals.

Most health coaching education programs include training in a range of dietary theories, so you shouldn't feel intimidated by reaching out to a coach because your eating habits don't fit neatly into a box. Seek out a coach who understands the concept of bio-individuality—the belief that there isn't one, single diet that's universally best for everyone—and you'll be off to a great start. The best health coaches keep an open mind when it comes to assessing their clients' personal needs, food preferences, health, and performance goals; and to tailoring their support and guidance accordingly.

I hope that the information provided in this book will inspire and empower you to move toward lasting health and optimal performance with curiosity, courage, and confidence. Have a reason for the things that you choose to do—or not to do. And don't hesitate to ask for some guidance if and when you need it.

Appendix One

Making Sustainable Food Choices

In the world of sports nutrition, the topic of how food is grown and where it comes from isn't routinely discussed. There may be some attention placed on the relative importance of any given food being organically grown, grass-fed, or pasture-raised. But just as food provides information to the body, it provides insights into the agricultural practices that are used to grow and transport it.

The next time you buy meat or pull a fruit or vegetable out of your refrigerator, give it a closer look. Where was it raised or grown? By who? How far did it travel to reach you?

We have all been told to read labels when we're selecting and purchasing food, which is good advice. But most sustainable foods don't have labels because they're fresh, whole, and unpackaged. In addition, sustainable foods don't harm the environment, are grown or raised with respect for both humans and animals, provide a fair wage to farmers, and support local economies instead of large corporations.

When making food choices, consider implementing at least a few of the following suggestions:

- **Eat locally grown foods.** Shop at your local farmer's market, join a CSA, or grow a few of your own vegetables in your backyard.
- **Eat seasonally grown foods.**
- **Instead of buying pre-prepared foods, make your own**—anything from taco seasoning, yogurt, and pesto to bone broth, granola, and pasta sauce.
- **Be willing to trade some time and convenience for honest-to-goodness food.** Prepare your meals at home. This may mean eating more simply, prioritizing the flavor (and nutrient density) of fewer ingredients.
- **Buy fair-trade.** If you don't know the source of your food because it's coming from another country, look for the words "fair-trade" on the label. They are sourced from producers who treat and pay their farmers well.
- **Consider the big picture before making value-based food judgments.** Buying locally and humanely raised animal products can be more sustainable than the foreign-grown grains and beans found in the bulk section of your natural food store.

Appendix Two

Building a Better Food Pyramid

Eating well doesn't require following a limited or regimented diet. It's more about establishing a satisfying and sustainable balance of the right types (and relative amounts) of food that support your health and performance goals.

It's also important to realize that the health-enhancing benefits of any given food strategy often stem more from what you don't eat than what you do.

Begin by eating the FOUNDATIONAL FOODS described below. They provide the broad base of critical nutrients a woman's body needs to thrive. This simple, basic diet nourished and sustained our primitive ancestors for millennia. Since our underlying genetics haven't really changed, satisfy your body's most fundamental nutrients needs by making these foods the largest part of your diet:

Non-starchy vegetables, especially leafy greens such as mustard or collard; kale, watercress, bok choy, spinach, broccoli rabe, napa cabbage, Brussels sprouts, Swiss chard and arugula. In an effort to limit your exposure to thallium and other toxins found in fracking brine, do your best to avoid eating leafy greens grown in the state of California.

Animal proteins. Favor ruminants—animals that feed on grass and leaves (beef, lamb, bison, elk, venison, goat). When it comes to beef, buy grass-fed and pasture-raised and choose the fattier cuts. Eat pork, turkey, and chicken with more moderation (they are higher in omega-6 fats). Opt for wild, line-caught fish and fertile or pastured organic eggs.

Fermented foods. Sauerkraut and kimchi; pickled beets and vegetables; fermented liquids such as kefir and kombucha.

Sea vegetables. Arame, dulse, wakame, nori, and hijiki are a few tasty examples. Look for Maine Sea Coast products, which are not sourced from the potentially radioactive waters off the coast of Japan.

Healthy, unprocessed fats and oils. Coconut, avocado, olive, macadamia, and red palm (from a family owned farm or other sustainable source); butter and lard from organic, grass-fed, free-range cattle. These oils can be used for sustained energy and higher-heat cooking except for macadamia and olive oils, which can both withstand low heat but are better thought of as foods.

Natural, elemental salt. Use North, Mediterranean, Hawaiian, or Celtic sea salts; Himalayan or Real® crystal salts only. Strictly avoid table salt.

Teas. Herbal, green, black, and white; yerba mate. For a hot or cold instant alternative, try Wisdom of the Ancients *Yerba Mate Royale* (available at vitacost.com)

Add some diversity to your diet by eating SUPPORTIVE FOODS, which should be viewed as secondary sources of nutrition. These foods add nutrient-rich variety (and practical convenience) to life, but are best when used to supplement your intake of Foundational Foods.

Protein powders. Hydrolyzed beef protein powder offers the most complete amino acid profile for growth, repair, and recovery (and it tastes great). Good plant-based sources include hemp, pea, and pumpkin seed powders.

A powdered fruit, vegetable, and herbal concentrate like *Chocoberry Blast*™ (available on Amazon or at purecleanperformance.com). This chocolate superfood blend not only provides a broad base of nutrient support, but improves the flavor of any protein-based smoothie or blended drink.

Non-dairy milks. Coconut, hemp seed, and nut milks are all good choices. For a more nutrient-rich, cost-effective, and environmentally sound alternative to aseptic packages, make your own non-dairy milk at home. There are dozens of made-from-scratch recipes available on the internet. You can substitute unsweetened coconut flakes or chips in any recipe using nuts when making coconut milk. There are a number of coconut milk powders (that blend easily with water) available, too. Look for a brand that is casein and maltodextrin free.

Blending water with nut butter may yield the most waste-free and nutrient-rich milk. And it offers you the ability to make as much—or as little—milk as you need at any given time. If you're buying pre-packaged, *Tempt* (hemp), *Ripple* (yellow pea), and *Vita Coco* (coconut) milks are the most nutrient-dense options to choose from.

Fruits and berries. Small amounts of those in season.

Nuts. Including Brazil nuts, pine nuts, chestnuts, hazelnuts, walnuts, macadamias, almonds, cashews, and pistachios; all preferably raw.

Seeds. Chia, hemp, pumpkin, sunflower, sesame, and flax.

Root vegetables. Red beets, carrots, parsnips, squashes, turnips, rutabagas, radishes, jicama, Jerusalem artichokes, heirloom potatoes, sweet potatoes, and yams.

Use caution when eating SUPPORTIVE FOODS WITH LIMITS. Supportive foods are still relatively nutrient-rich but tend to be allergenic and/or high in insulin-spiking carbohydrates. Their intake should be more infrequent.

Grass-fed whey protein powder, preferably from goat milk. Mt. Capra offers a variety of great-tasting, highly digestible, and hypoallergenic grass-fed goat proteins. They are available on Amazon or at Vitacost.com.

Raw, organic dairy or cheese products made from cow, goat, or sheep's milk. According to Dr. Josh Axe (and many other functional medicine specialists), an extensive look into research and claims made by the U.S. Food and Drug Administration and Centers for Disease Control related to raw milk being dangerous have been found to be completely unwarranted. In fact, consuming pasteurized milk products is potentially more problematic since they come from cows raised in concentrated animal feeding operations (CAFOs), which are the perfect breeding ground for foodborne illnesses.

Raw milk is rich in minerals and healthy bacteria that can benefit your digestive system. It also contains a variety of enzymes that can help improve the digestion of nutrients from other foods.

Organic, grass-fed, and whole-fat yogurts, which can sometimes be difficult to find in grocery stores but can be made easily and inexpensively at home.

Complex, grain-based carbohydrates, including small amounts of wild rice (a grass), amaranth and teff (which are both high in protein), millet, quinoa, and buckwheat (which are actually seeds). Experiment with eliminating all other grains (especially wheat) from your diet. Many women have enjoyed improvements in their overall health and wellbeing from going both gluten and grain-free.

Oils high in PUFA (polyunsaturated fat), including flax, walnut, and sesame which should not be used during cooking but can add an occasional and enjoyable burst of flavor to any dish or salad.

Reduce or eliminate your intake of LIMITED FOODS, which have been traditionally eaten around the world because they offer an inexpensive source of calories. Limited foods are inherently low in nutrient value and contain mild toxins that, when eaten frequently, can lead to or exacerbate inflammatory conditions that interfere with the body's performance capacity and healing process.

When FOUNDATIONAL and SUPPORTIVE foods are readily available, LIMITED foods should be removed from your diet entirely.

White potatoes, especially Idaho and russet. Since white potatoes have a higher glycemic index, opt for waxy varieties including red bliss or new potatoes. Yukon gold, red fingerlings and/or heirloom varieties are also good choices. Cooking and cooling potatoes before they are eaten restructures them into a resistant starch, which reduces their total carbohydrate content and makes them an excellent prebiotic (food source for beneficial intestinal bacteria).

Keep in mind that white potatoes are also a *nightshade*, a member of the plant family Solanaceae which includes eggplant, tomatoes, and peppers (although black pepper is a different plant). While most women can safely consume these vegetables without any inflammatory consequences, those who suffer from arthritis, joint pain, and/or an autoimmune disease often feel and perform better without them.

Legumes. All bean varieties including peanuts.

Grains, including those that are marketed as healthier varieties of wheat—emmer, einkorn, farro, kamut, spelt, wheat germ, and wheat berries. If you must eat grains, choose those that are sprouted, organic, and gluten-free. Opt for white over brown rice (since it contains less arsenic and fewer anti-nutrients) and steel-cut over rolled oats (since their glycemic index is much lower).

If it's NOT FOOD, don't eat it.

What's inside the boxes and bags found on grocery store shelves might be marketed and sold to us as food, but these products of modern industry are not what they appear to be. While refined and processed products may provide calories, they do so to the detriment of our overall health. Strictly avoid eating the following food-like substances:

Conventional processed and/or packaged meats. The quality of the meat you eat is important. Organic, grass-fed, pasture-raised products are far superior to those from CAFOs which are likely to be contaminated with herbicides, pesticides, hormones, antibiotics (and other drugs), as well as genetically modified organisms from the artificially engineered grains these animals are fed.

In 2009, a joint research project between the U.S. Department of Agriculture and Clemson University determined that when compared to grain-fed, grass-fed beef is not only higher in total omega-3's with a much healthier omega-6 to omega-3 ratio, but higher in B and E vitamins, beta carotene, calcium, magnesium, and potassium.

Refined and processed sugars. White beet sugar, corn syrup and corn syrup solids, barley malt, dehydrated cane juice, cane juice solids and crystals, turbinado, date sugar, glucose, sucrose, fructose, and dextrose. Refined sugars are not only pervasive in all types of candies, sweetened beverages (including bottled smoothies, coffees, and teas), jams, jellies, and baked goods, flavored milks and yogurts, condiments and sauces, 'sports' drinks, soups, cereals, cereal bars, and canned goods.

Artificial colors, flavors (including MSG), sweeteners, and preservatives.

Processed, hydrogenated oils. Don't be fooled into thinking vegetable oils are healthy. They're extracted from seeds with poisonous solvents (like hexane). In addition to being inherently toxic and easily damaged by heat, vegetable oils are overloaded with omega-6 fats. Strictly avoid the use of canola, corn, soybean, grape seed, cottonseed, safflower, sunflower, and peanut oils. When you eat out, ask what kind of oil is being used to prepare your meal. Even the finest restaurants use vegetable oils (especially corn and soy) in their kitchens.

Refined and processed grains, which represent the majority of SAD (Standard American Diet), packaged foods found in the middle aisles and frozen section of the grocery store. They include all products made from grain-based flours—breads, pastas, cereals, crackers, chips, and baked goods.

Instead of eating (or baking with) refined grains, explore and experiment with the wide variety of gluten-free, grain-free (nut), or resistant-starch-based flours (such as plantain, potato, and cassava) that are now readily available. In the snack and pasta sections, look for the bean-based products that are becoming more widely available. Although beans are not an ideal source of nutrients and calories, they are superior to grains.

Soy, with the exception of occasional tempeh, miso, and natto (organic), which are made from fermented soy.

GMO foods. Unfortunately, the list of genetically modified foods is growing but primarily includes corn, soy, canola, zucchini, yellow squash, papaya, and sugar beets. See Chapter Seven for information on how to identify GMO foods by their PLU code.

Alcohol, excepting small amounts of red (preferably dry-farmed, organic, and sulfite-free) wine.

It's fine to add a little FLAVOR to your life. While these items aren't considered foods because they don't provide the body with measurable amounts of macronutrients, they still offer several documented health and performance benefits.

Dark chocolate. Fair-trade, sustainable, and greater than 70% cocoa content.

Coffee. Look for single-bean, water-processed Arabica beans that have been shade grown at high altitudes. This type of coffee is preferable because of its low mycotoxin (mold) content. I can personally recommend Lifeboost™ beans (available at lifeboost.com).

Natural, unrefined sweeteners. Stevia, raw coconut sugar, raw honey, yacon and grade B maple syrups, monk fruit powder or syrup. Sugar alcohols including erythritol, xylitol, and maltitol (in small amounts). Avoid the use of refined sweeteners being sold as 'healthy' sugar alternatives such as agave nectar, brown rice syrup, barley malt, turbinado, date sugar, and evaporated cane juice solids.

Herbs and spices. The variety of choices is endless—and exciting!

Appendix Three

Using Targeted Nutritional Supplements

While nutritional supplements may be a billion dollar industry, it's better to spend your hard-earned money buying fresh, nutrient-rich foods. Since the human body is hardwired to thrive on whole foods, rely more on what you eat—as opposed to what supplements you take—for optimal health, performance, and recovery. Having said that, there are a few important nutrients that can be difficult to obtain significantly and consistently from food alone and/or may be needed in larger amounts when recovering from an illness or injury.

Dietary supplements to consider include:

- **A phytonutrient-rich food supplement.** Look for a nutrient-rich, alkalizing formula with plenty of antioxidant-rich fruits and vegetables. A high-quality formula like *Chocoberry Blast*™ from PureClean Performance (purecleanperformance.com) will also contain herbal concentrates to support efficient liver detoxification, good gastrointestinal health, high nitric oxide levels, and reduced inflammation.

- **An essential fatty acid formula.** Optimal and balanced levels of essential fatty acids are critical for optimal health, performance, and recovery. Laboratory assessments have shown that most women need about 2,400 mg of EPA/DHA from a trusted fish oil source to achieve optimal omega-3 levels. If you have already been supplementing your diet with an omega-3 fatty acid formula, it's essential to check your blood levels on a regular basis to make sure that your omega-3 index stays between 10 and 12%. Recent research has shown that omega-3 fatty acids make muscles more receptive to training stimuli.

- **A highly absorbable form of vitamin D3** in conjunction with at least 100ug of vitamin K2 (which synergistically supports the absorption and beneficial actions of vitamin D3) daily.

Due to a chronic lack of sunshine and the overuse of sunscreens, research suggests that almost 85% of the U.S. population is deficient in vitamin D3. This is a serious problem since it's one of the most important nutrients in the body. Vitamin D3 is not only a building block of the entire endocrine system, it supports the body's immune response and regulates bone, brain, and cardiovascular health. It has also been shown to shorten the duration of illness and injury, increase muscle strength, enhance reaction time, and improve both coordination and balance.

Laboratory assessments suggest that most women will need to take at least 5,000 iu of vitamin D3 daily and, when possible, get 15-20 minutes of full-body exposure to direct, mid-day sunlight two to three times a week. If you begin taking a vitamin D3 supplement, make sure to assess your blood level after four months. Adjust your intake accordingly in order to maintain a blood level between 55 and 65 pg/ml.

- **An essential amino acid formula.** Even when your diet includes adequate amounts of plant and animal protein, your body may still require a larger supply of essential amino acids to build strength, create energy, and repair completely. Age, stress, and poor digestion all interfere with dietary protein digestion and utilization. If you suffer from frequent muscle, tendon, or joint injuries, fatigue or poor recovery, 20 grams of a high-quality essential amino acid formula taken daily may provide your body with the additional support it needs.

  I recommend *FundAminos*™ essential amino acid blend from PureClean Performance (purecleanperformance.com). This 100% natural, plant-based essential amino acid product is physician-formulated and has been receiving consistently positive reviews from athletes for more than a decade.

- **A readily absorbed magnesium supplement.** Since minerals play a key role in hundreds of physiological processes, they are just as important to the body as water and air. Magnesium contributes directly to energy production, supports healthy adrenal function, and promotes optimum muscular, skeletal, cardiovascular, and hormonal health. It also calms the nervous system, improving the quality of sleep. Because most of the magnesium we consume in food is destroyed by the process of digestion, the use of a topical (rub-on or soak-in) formula is an effective strategy for restoring and rebalancing the body's stores. I can personally recommend the Ancient Minerals product line (ancient-minerals.com).

Appendix Four

The Abbreviated Guide to Identifying and Minimizing Toxins

Toxins are poisonous substances (either natural or synthetic) that actively promote chronic inflammation and a general state of dis-ease throughout the body. A list of the most common toxins and their sources follows below.

Toxins Found in Food and Water

Processed and heated vegetable oils. The most pervasive offenders are soy, canola, and corn oils, which are all hydrogenated and easily damaged by heat. These are the most common oils used in commercially fried foods. Due to their poor fatty acid profiles, avoid grape seed, cotton seed, safflower, sunflower, and peanut oils as well.

Meats and starches cooked at high temperatures. Choose longer, low-heat cooking methods over broiling or grilling.

Genetically Modified Organisms (GMOs). The most commonly modified plants have had an insecticide gene implanted into their

DNA which makes them more pest-resistant. The most frequently reported health problems associated with the consumption of GMOs are gastrointestinal disorders and immune dysfunction. See Chapter Seven for information on how to identify GMO foods by their PLU code.

Unfermented soy products. They contain large amounts of phytoestrogens (plant estrogens) which promote fat production and contribute to hormonal imbalances in both men and women. They also contain enzyme inhibitors, which interfere with protein digestion and haemagglutinin, a glycoprotein (a protein with a sugar attached to it) which causes red blood cells to clump together hindering oxygen uptake. Because its underlying amino acid structure is imbalanced, the body has a difficult time digesting and utilizing unfermented soy. This makes it a poor source of dietary protein.

Fermented soy products like natto, tempeh, and miso, however, are low in the anti-nutrients that prevent the absorption of minerals like calcium, magnesium, iron, and zinc. They're also easier to digest. In fact, they contain friendly bacteria (probiotics) that can improve digestion and increase nutrient absorption. Fermented soy products are high in vitamin K2, which support bone and cardiovascular health.

Artificial sweeteners. Saccharin, acesulfame, aspartame, neotame, and sucralose. Use stevia (an herb) as a non-caloric alternative. Or better yet, opt for raw honey, coconut sugar, maple syrup, molasses, or unrefined cane sugar. While these sweeteners do contain calories, they also offer beneficial nutrients. Research done on the use of artificial (zero-calorie) sweeteners and weight management shows that they offer no measurable benefits. In fact, they have been linked to an increased risk of weight gain, obesity, high blood pressure, diabetes, heart disease, and other health problems.

MSG is an *excitotoxin* or nerve cell stimulant that has been linked to the onset of a variety of neurological disorders. MSG is commonly used as a flavor enhancer. While it's not an ingredient frequently found on food labels, watch for it disguised as a "natural flavor, spice, or hydrolyzed yeast extract."

Canned foods (especially those that are acidic) that do not have a BPA-free lining. The natural acids these foods contain break down the can, allowing both chemicals and metals to be released.

Synthetic vitamins, especially antioxidants. Synthetic vitamins are generally not well-recognized or utilized by the body (because they are not food). As a result, they aren't very effective and can sometimes be harmful. The use of antioxidant vitamins are a particular concern. Antioxidants are only effective when they work together as a team with the companion nutrients they are found with in fresh, whole foods. Unless you have an identified deficiency, avoid the use of isolated vitamin C, vitamin E, and beta carotene supplements as these nutrients can create physiological imbalances which, in turn, promote chronic inflammation.

Fluoridated water. Silicoflourides are an industrial waste product that is routinely added to our water supply as a supplement to make our teeth stronger and less prone to cavities. While the topical fluoride found in toothpaste can be beneficial, drinking fluoride to protect our teeth is a lot like swallowing sunscreen to protect our skin from sunburn. Fluoride exposure has been linked to a variety of health-related problems including bone and joint pain, immune disorders, and hormonal imbalances. Consider the use of a reverse osmosis filter for your drinking water if it comes from a fluoridated source.

Toxins Found in Personal Care Products

With an ever-increasing number of non-toxic cosmetics and personal care products available, it's becoming easier (and more affordable) to purchase chemical-free makeups, moisturizers, deodorants, shampoos, conditioners, and lipsticks.

Avoiding the use of any personal care products that remain on the skin for an extended period of time is particularly important. The longer the chemical toxins they contain remain in contact with the skin, the more completely they will be absorbed.

Pay Close Attention to the Dirty Dozen, which are the 12 most commonly identified toxins found in women's cosmetics and personal care products. According to recent research, one in eight of the 82,000 ingredients used in these products are industrial chemicals. Some of these are plasticizers (chemicals that keep concrete soft); others are degreasers (used to get grime off auto parts), and surfactants (they reduce surface tension in water, like those used in paints and inks). The complete list of the Dirty Dozen can be found on page 272.

In addition to avoiding the Dirty Dozen, make an effort to minimize your use of products that contain a man-made alcohol known as **propylene glycol**. Propylene glycol is a viscous, colorless liquid that attracts and absorbs water so it makes the skin appear more supple. As a result, it is one of the most widely used ingredients in cosmetics and facial cleansers, moisturizers, bath soaps, shampoos and conditioners, deodorants, and shaving creams.

In addition to its use as an additive in cosmetic and personal care products, propylene glycol can be found in food items such as beer, packaged baked goods, frozen dairy products, margarine, coffee, nuts, and soda. It is also used as an inactive ingredient in many over-the-counter and prescription drugs, like cough syrup. Regularly ingesting or absorbing large amounts of propylene glycol can have harmful effects on the heart, liver, and nervous system by disrupting the production of certain neurotransmitters.

Choose your deodorant or antiperspirant carefully. While conventional products work (deodorants by inhibiting the body's ability to naturally secrete toxins and antiperspirants by clogging the skin follicles to deter sweating), they remain in constant contact with your skin and contain:

- **Aluminum Compounds.** Which are used to clog your pores in order to prevent sweating. Aluminum exposure has been strongly linked to Alzheimer's disease and estrogen imbalance.
- **Triclosan.** A featured member of the Dirty Dozen, triclosan is classified as a pesticide by the U.S. Food and Drug Administration. It has been banned from use in soaps, but is still found in the majority of name-brand deodorants. It's used to kill bacteria when it comes in contact with your skin. When triclosan is combined with water it can create chloroform, a carcinogenic gas.
- **Propylene Glycol.** This pervasive, skin-irritating chemical can become toxic when used topically or consumed orally on a regular basis.
- **Ethanolamines including TEA and DEA.** Another group of known carcinogens that have been banned for use throughout Europe.

Look for personal care products manufactured by Aubrey Organics, Burt's Bees, Jason, Miessence, Pangea Organics, Planet Botanicals, Suki, Teressentials, and Weleda. They are all reliably toxin-free.

Toxins at Home

Conventional cleaning products are among the most toxic substances found in the home. While they can sometimes be more expensive, natural alternatives like those made by Seventh Generation, Common Good, Ecos, Better Life, and Ecover are worth the extra cost. Those who are budget-conscious may find that the old-fashioned predecessors to commercial cleaning supplies—lemon juice, baking soda, Borax®, and vinegar—work just as well. Dr. Bronner's makes a good, all-around soap for general house cleaning and *Murphy's Oil Soap* is great for hardwood floors.

If you must use a chemical cleaning solution, always ventilate the area you're working in. Turn on a vent fan and open two windows on either side of the house to create air flow. Allow moving air to move through your work area for at least an hour after you've finished cleaning—or until the smell of the cleaning product is completely gone.

Chlorine. Make an effort to limit your exposure to chlorine bleach as a general cleaning and washing agent. Consider the use of a chlorine filter on your home drinking and bathing water if your public water supply is chlorinated.

When it comes to doing laundry, opt for natural **detergents, fabric softeners, and dryer sheets.** Wash new clothing, bedding, and towels at least twice (to reduce your exposure to any toxic fabric finishes) before use.

Pay particular attention to **dry-cleaned and/or conventionally laundered clothing** since they both contain toxic chemical residues that remain in constant and direct contact with the skin.

Don't use conventional air fresheners and avoid synthetic fragrances. If a product is scented with anything but an essential oil, it is probably disrupting your hormones.

Replace vinyl shower curtains with those made of fabric and choose from toxin-free alternatives when it comes to using paint and installing floor and wall coverings in your home.

Discontinue the use of any aluminum or non-stick Teflon™ pots and pans. Aluminum has been linked to the onset of Alzheimer's disease; it can also harm the brain and bones. Perfluorooctanoic acid (PFOA) is a cancer-causing chemical used in the production of Teflon™. Stainless steel, cast iron, glass, and ceramic coated cast iron are the best materials for cooking. Use stainless steel utensils for eating. Don't bake food of any kind on aluminum foil. Instead, use unbleached parchment paper or bake directly on an aluminum and PFOA-free pan. Avoid drinking out of aluminum water bottles.

Be wary of any glass or ceramic drink or dinnerware made in China. While they are considered 'food safe' by the U.S. Food and Drug Administration, the glazes used on these products often contain lead and/or cadmium. These toxins can leach into your food, especially when heated. When looking for dinnerware that's free of lead and cadmium, consider unglazed, high-fired porcelain or stoneware.

Styrofoam plates, bowls, or cups should never be used. They contain BPA and/or BPS which can leach into food and water, hot or cold.

Store food in glass, not plastic. Stock up on glass storage containers (recycled glass jars or mason jars can work well for many things).

Because plastic is unbreakable, there may be an occasional time and place for it. But never eat food or drink liquids that have been heated in plastic. (even by the sun). Never store any kind of acidic food or beverage (such as pineapple or orange juice, tomatoes, or items that contain vinegar) in a plastic container. If you must use plastic, look for items imprinted with the HDPE #2 or #4 'chasing arrows' symbol.

Don't forget to use non-toxic pest control methods in your garden and avoid using toxic flea shampoos, collars, and other related pesticides on your pets.

Appendix Five

Resources

Professional Organizations

http://www.acam.org
The American College for Advancement in Medicine is the leading Integrative Medicine organization in the world. Integrative Medicine combines conventional and alternative therapies to improve patient care. Rather than practicing one type of medicine, integrative physicians will often combine therapies and treatment approaches to ensure the best results for their patients. While ACAM physicians use western medicine, they also embrace and incorporate any proven and appropriate alternative treatment options.

https://afmassociation.com
The American Functional Medicine Association (AFMA) is a non-profit organization comprised of scientists and healthcare practitioners ranging from physicians, pharmacists, scientists, and naturopaths to chiropractors, nurses, midwives, and physician assistants. The organization's mission is to promote the science of integrative medicine, provide cutting edge science-based conferences, and improve the practice of both medicine and patient care.

https://aofm.org
The Association of Functional Medicine's core purpose is to educate prospective patients about the benefits of functional medicine. The organization achieves this through a variety of web based assessments tools and connection platforms that bring doctors and patients together.

https://aanmc.org
The American Association of Naturopathic Physicians actively supports, promotes, and advocates on behalf of naturopathic physicians. The organization's expressed goal is, "to transform the health care system from disease management to health promotion by incorporating the principles of naturopathic medicine."

Books

The Primal Blueprint **by Mark Sisson**
This best-selling book is often referred to as the primal health and wellness 'bible.' *The Primal Blueprint* catapulted the ancestral health movement into the mainstream and launched a nutrition and lifestyle program that has helped tens of thousands of people reach their health and fitness goals. In this book, author Mark Sisson dispels many of the dietary myths we've been led to believe over the past 30 years.

It Starts with Food: Discover the Whole30 and Change Your Life in Unexpected Ways **by Dallas Harwig**
This transformative, 30-day program offers a clear, balanced, and sustainable plan for changing the way you eat and improving the overall quality of your life in profound, lasting, and unexpected ways. Since 2009, the *Whole30* program has quietly introduced thousands of people to a healthier relationship with

food. Think of this program as an opportunity to hit your nutritional 'reset button.'

Perfect Health Diet by Paul Jaminet, Ph.D.
Suffering from chronic illness and unable to get satisfactory results from doctors, husband and wife scientists Paul and Shou-Ching Jaminet took an intensely personal interest in health and nutrition. They embarked on five years of rigorous research. What they found changed their lives—and the lives of thousands of their readers. Their ancestral-based work combines insights from evolutionary biology and an overview of current nutritional literature to offer an innovative view of the optimal human diet.

ROAR: How to Match Your Food and Fitness to Your Unique Female Physiology for Optimum Performance, Great Health, and a Strong, Lean Body for Life by Stacy Simms and Selene Yeager
ROAR is a comprehensive, physiology-based nutrition and training guide specifically designed for active women. This book provides practical insights on how to adapt your nutrition, hydration, and training to fit your unique, female physiology.

Practical Paleo by Diane Sanflippo, BS, NC
A goldmine of information for anyone who wants to focus on improving their digestive health. Diane's book is especially useful for anyone seeking a broad and well-balanced introduction to the paleo diet—and for anyone searching for new ideas on how to fine-tune their health and performance food strategy. *Practical Paleo* offers a customized approach to the healthy, whole-food lifestyle.

The Craving Brain by Ronald Ruden, MD
A fascinating read on the innate, physiological reactions that originate in and continue to drive our primitive brain. In his book, Dr.

Ruden asserts that the roots of addiction do not lie in our character, but in the complex chain reaction that originates in an ancient survival mechanism in the brain.

Healthy Gut, Healthy You by Michael Ruscio, D.C
If you are living with depression, fatigue, a thyroid imbalance, joint pain, insomnia, or chronic inflammation; gas, bloating, diarrhea, constipation, or abdominal pain, your symptoms could be caused by a bacterial imbalance in your gut. In *Healthy Gut, Healthy You*, clinician and researcher Dr. Michael Ruscio reveals how modern lifestyle changes and the widespread use of antibiotics has made us more vulnerable to illness and injury than ever before.

The Kaufman Protocol: Why We Age and How to Stop It by Sandra Kaufman, M.D.
Dr. Kaufman's book brings the science of aging out of the laboratory and into the real world where it can be easily and practically implemented. The first half of the book discusses cellular aging; the second provides a clear overview of the top 15 nutrients and supplements that can be used to curtail it. A must-read for anyone interested in the rapidly expanding field of anti-aging medicine.

Podcasts

Revolution Radio with Chris Kresser, LAc
Bulletproof Radio with Dave Asprey
Primal Diet, Modern Health with Beverly Meyer, CCN
Myers Way with Amy Myers, MD
ThePaleo Solution with Rob Wolfe
Balanced Bites: Modern Healthy Living with Diane Sanfilippo CN & Liz Wolfe NTP

Websites and Blogs

http://www.marksdailyapple.com
One of the top resources on the internet for everything you wanted to know about living a longer, healthier, and more productive life.

https://www.drruscio.com
Gut health and healthy digestion are arguably the foundation of good overall health. Recent research has drawn a connection between the health of your stomach and intestines and that of your brain, heart, immune system, and your ability to absorb the nutrients that fuel optimal health, performance, and recovery. Visit Dr. Ruscio's site and explore his many popular articles on the topic of gut health.

https://www.elitehrv.com
The global leader in heart rate variability for health improvement and sports performance optimization.

https://www.heartmath.com
A proven program using HRV technology to help you reduce stress and anxiety by reclaiming your inner balance. Heartmath is based on 26 years of research and is recommended by thousands of health care professionals.

http://www.chriskresser.com
A national leader in the field of functional medicine, Chris is a great resource for any health or performance concern.

http://www.balancedbites.com
Diane Sanflippo's online site picks up where her book, *Practical Paleo*, leaves off. A wide variety of podcasts and articles about

different health conditions and concerns are available. Diane's insightful suggestions are both simple and sustainable.

https://wellnessmama.com
A trusted, online resource for health-minded women. The website covers a variety of health, parenting, and natural living topics, summarizing information in a clear and usable way. Visit wellnessmama.com for practical health tips, real-food recipes, DIY beauty instructions, green cleaning tutorials, natural remedies, and other useful information that can make your life simpler, healthier, and happier.

Links for Food Lovers

http://www.primal-palate.com
http://www.health-bent.com
http://www.paleodietlifestyle.com
http://www.chowstalker.com
http://www.paleorecipes.chriskresser.com
http://www.paleorecipebook.com
http://www.paleomg.com
http://www.paleoleap.com
http://www.wholekitchensink.com

Selected Bibliography

American Journal of Clinical Nutrition. 2006 April; 83(4): 941S–944S. **Status of nutrition education in medical schools.** Kelly Adams, et al.

Current Gastrointestinal Reports. 2013; 15(12): 356. **Gas and the Microbiome.** M. Pimentel, et al.

Global Advances in Health Medicine. 2013 July; 2(4): 38–57. **A Systematic Review of the Literature on Health and Wellness Coaching: Defining a Key Behavioral Variable in Intervention in Healthcare.** Ruth Q. Wolever, PhD, et al.

Running Research News. 2005 April 22; **Science of Sport: The Gender Gap.** Owen Anderson.

Medicine and Science in Sports and Exercise. 2010 October; 42(10): 64-65. **AR1 Estrogen Loss Leads to Reduced Motor Activity: Neural versus Muscular Role?** Helder Fonseca, et al.

Sports Medicine. 1993 December; 16(6): 400-430. **Effect of Different Phases of the Menstrual Cycle and Oral Contraceptives on Athletic Performance.** Constance Lebrun.

American Journal of Clinical Nutrition. 2000; 72(4): 946-953. **Energy Metabolism after Two Years of Energy Restriction: The Biosphere 2 Experiment.** C. Weyer, et al.

European Journal of Applied Physiology. 2014 January; 114(1): 93-103. **Effects of Probiotic Supplementation on Gastrointestinal Permeability, Inflammation and Exercise Performance in the Heat.** Cecilia Shing, et al.

American Journal of Public Health. 1997; 87: 992-997. **Milk, Dietary Calcium, and Bone Fractures in Women: A 12-Year Prospective Study.** D. Feskanich, et al.

American Journal of Clinical Nutrition. 2006 October; 84(4): 936-942. **Colas, but not Other Beverages, are Associated with Low Bone Mineral Density in Older Women: The Framingham Osteoporosis Study.** L. Appel, et al.

HowStuffWorks.com. 2008 October 8; **Do Men and Women Have Different Brains?** Molly Edmonds.

Nutrition Review. 1992; 50: 3. **The Role of Dietary Fatty Acids in Biology: Their Place in the Evolution of the Human Brain.** M. Crawford.

Critical Review of Food Science and Nutrition. 2009; 49: 327-360. **Gastrointestinal Effects of Low-Digestible Carbohydrates.** H. Grabitske, J. Slavin.

An Evidence-Based Approach to Vitamins and Minerals. 2003. Linus Pauling Institute. J. Higdon.

Journal of the International Society of Sports Nutrition. 2006; 3: 51-55. **Food Alone May Not Provide Sufficient Micronutrients for Preventing Deficiency.** B. Misner.

Extreme Physiology and Medicine. 2014; 3: 18. **Are We Being Drowned in Hydration Advice?** J. Cotter.

European Journal of Sports Science. 2014 April 25; 14(8): 847-851. **Where are all the female participants in Sports and Exercise Medicine research?** J. Costello, et al.

Natural Products Insider. 2018 June; 8(12): 7-13. **The Goldilocks Issue: When Will Sports Nutrition Fit Women Just Right?** Steve Myers.

Alternative Medical Review. 1999 August; 4(4): 249-265. **Nutritional and Botanical Interventions to Assist with the Adaptation to Stress.** G. Kelly.

The Paleo Diet for Athletes. 2005. Rodale Press. Loren Cordain and Joe Friel.

Sports Science Exchange. 1995; 58(8): 5. **The Role of Meat in an Athlete's Diet: Its Effect on Key Macro and Micronutrients.** Susan Kleiner.

British Journal of Nutrition. 2009 December; 102(12): 1803-10. **Relationship Between Animal Protein Intake and Muscle Mass Index in Healthy Women**. M. Aubertin-Leheudre and H. Adlercreutz.

Biomedical Pharmacotherapy. 2002 October; 56(8): 365-379. **The Importance of the Ratio of Omega 6/Omega 3 Essential Fatty Acids**. A. Simopoulos.

Journal of the Academy of Nutrition and Dietetics. 2012 April; 4: 548-552. **Whole Beetroot Consumption Acutely Improves Running Performance**. M. Murphy, et al.

Journal of Applied Physiology. 2010 November 1; 109(5): 1394-1403. **Acute L-Arginine Supplementation Reduces the O_2 Cost of Moderate-Intensity Exercise and Enhances High-Intensity Exercise Tolerance**. S.J. Bailey, et al.

American Journal of Public Health. 1997; 87: 992-997. **Milk, Dietary Calcium, and Bone Fractures in Women: A 12-Year Prospective Study**. D. Feskanich, et al.

Nutrition Guide for Clinicians, 1st edition. 2007. Physician's Committee for Responsible Medicine. N. Barnard, et al.

Advanced Nutrition and Human Metabolism, 3rd edition. 1999. Delmar Publishers, Inc. J. Groff and S. Gropper.

European Journal of Clinical Nutrition. 2014; 68: 641. **Beyond Weight Loss: A Review of the Therapeutic Uses of Very-Low-Carbohydrate (Ketogenic) Diets**. A Paoli, et al.

Applied Physiology for Nutrition and Metabolism. 2015; 40: 755-761. **Protein: A Nutrient in Focus**. E. Arentson, et al.

International Journal of Sports Nutrition and Exercise Metabolism. 2016; 16: 129-152. **A Review of Issues: Dietary Protein Intake in Humans**. S. Bilsborough and N. Mann.

https://www.epa.gov. 2016. **Federal Research on Recycled Tire Crumb Used on Playing Fields.** *The Environmental Protection Agency.* Washington, DC.

Sports Health. January/February 2019. doi: 10.1177/1941738118793378. **Synthetic Turf: History, Design, Maintenance, and Athlete Safety.** J.R. Jastifer, et al.

International Journal of Oncology. August 2017; 51(2): 405–413. **World Health Organization, Radiofrequency Radiation and Health—A Hard Nut to Crack.** Lennart Hardell.

Food and Agriculture Organization for the United Nations. 2011. **Dietary Protein Quality Evaluation in Human Nutrition.** Auckland, NZ.

International Anesthesiology Clinics. 2007 Spring; 45(2): 27-37. **Cytokines, Inflammation, and Pain.** Jun-Ming Zhang, M.D. and Jianxiong An, M.D.

http://chriskresser.com. 2013 April 26; **The Diet-Heart Myth: Why Everyone Should Know Their LDL Particle Number.** Chris Kresser.

American Journal of Clinical Nutrition. 2004; 79: 899S. **Is a Calorie a Calorie?** A. Buchholz and D. Schoeller.

Sports Medicine. 2010 January 1; 40(1); 41-58. **The Influence of Estrogen on Skeletal Muscle: Sex Matters.** D.L. Enns and P.M. Tiidus.

Orthopedic Clinics of North America. 2006; 37: 575. **Female Athlete Triad and Stress Fractures.** D. Feingold and S. Hame.

Amino Acids. 2009 May; 37(1): 1-17. **Amino Acids: Metabolism, Functions, and Nutrition.** G. Wu.

Nutrition and Metabolism. 2005 September; 2: 25. **Dietary Protein Intake and Renal Function.** W. Martin, et al.

American Journal of Clinical Nutrition. 2003 October; 78(4): 734-741. **An Increase in Dietary Protein Improves the Blood Glucose Response in Persons with Type 2 Diabetes.** M. Gannon, et al.

PLOS One. 2010 August 11; 5(8): 121-122. **Dietary Protein and Blood Pressure: A Systematic Review.** W. Altorf-van der Kuil, et al.

American Journal of Clinical Nutrition. 2005 July; 82(1): 41-48. **A High-Protein Diet Induces Sustained Reductions in Appetite, Ad Libitum Caloric Intake, and Body Weight Despite Compensatory Changes in Diurnal Plasma Leptin and Ghrelin Concentrations.** D. Weigle, et al.

Journal of Bone and Mineral Research. 2009 December 2; Published online. **Dietary Protein and Bone Health.** René Rizzoli and Jean-Philippe Bonjour.

Current Opinions in Lipidology. 2011 February 22; (1): 16-20. **Dietary Protein and Skeletal Health: A Review of Recent Human Research.** J. Kerstetter, et al.

American Journal of Clinical Nutrition. 1999 January; 69(1): 147-152. **Prospective Study of Dietary Protein Intake and Risk of Hip Fracture in Postmenopausal Women.** R. Munger, et al.

Journal of the American Medical Association. 2005 November 16; 294(19): 2455-2464. **Effects of Protein, Monounsaturated Fat, and Carbohydrate Intake on Blood Pressure and Serum Lipids: Results of the OmniHeart Randomized Trial.** Lawrence Appel, et al.

The American Journal of Clinical Nutrition, 2015 March 1; 1(3): 496–505. **Effect of Protein Overfeeding on Energy Expenditure Measured in a Metabolic Chamber.** George Bray, et al.

Critical Review of Food Science and Nutrition. 2009; 49: 327-360. **Gastrointestinal Effects of Low-Digestible Carbohydrates.** H. Grabitske and J. Slavin.

The Best Things You Can Eat. 2013. Da Capo Lifelong Books. D. Grotto.

An Evidence-Based Approach to Vitamins and Minerals. 2003. Linus Pauling Institute. J. Higdon.

www.consumerreports.org. **Arsenic in Your Food.** Published online 2012

Annual Review of Plant Biology. 2013; 16: 19-46. **Plants, Diet, and Health.** C. Martin.

Diabetes, Obesity, and Metabolism. 2002 January 4; **Effects of Water-Soluable Extract of Maitake Mushroom on Circulating Glucose/Insulin Concentrations in KK Mice.** V. Manohar, et al.

Nutrition and Cancer. 2008; 60(6): 744-756. **White Button Mushroom Exhibits Antiproliferative and Proapoptotic Properties and Inhibits Prostate Tumor Growth in Athymic Mice.** L. Adams, et al.

BioMed Research International. 2016 November 29; 1(50): 39-56. **Effect of 48-Hour Fasting on Autonomic Function, Brain Activity, Cognition, and Mood in Amateur Weight Lifters.** R. Solianik, et al.

Journal of the International Society of Sports Nutrition. 2006; 3: 51-55. **Food Alone May Not Provide Sufficient Micronutrients for Preventing Deficiency.** B. Misner.

Journal of the American Medical Association. 2012 June 27; 307(24): 2627-2634. **Effects of Dietary Composition on Energy Expenditure During Weight-Loss Maintenance.**

Nutrition Bulletin. 2005; 30: 27-54. **Health Properties of Resistant Starch.** British Nutrition Foundation. A. Nugent.

Eating on the Wild Side. 2013. Little, Brown and Company. J. Robinson.

American Journal Obstetrics and Gynecology. 1982. March 15; 142(6.2): 735-738. **Metabolic Effects of Progesterone.** R. Kalkhoff.

Extreme Physiology and Medicine. 2014; 3: 18. **Are We Being Drowned in Hydration Advice?** J. Cotter.

Perfect Health Diet. 2012. Scribner Publishing. Paul Jaminet.

Nutrition and Health. 2000; 14(4): 195-204. **Field Studies on the Effects of Food Content on Wakefulness.** U. Landström, et al.

American Journal of Medicine. 2006 December; 119(12): 1005–1012. **Valerian Root for Sleep: A Systematic Review and Meta-Analysis.** Stephen Bent, MD, et al.

Journal of Clinical Endocrinology and Metabolism. 2005 September; 90(9): 5483-5488. **The Evidence for a Narrower Thyrotropin Reference Range is Compelling.** L. Wartofsky, et al.

Journal of Clinical Endocrinology and Metabolism. 2004 October; 87(3): 1068-1072. **Narrow Individual Variations in Serum T4 and T3 in the Normal Subjects: A Clue to the Understanding of Subclinical Thyroid Disease.** A. Stig, et al.

Psychoneuroendocrinology. 2015 September; 59: 25–36. **Distinct Cognitive Effects of Estrogen and Progesterone in Menopausal Women.** A. Berent-Spillson, et al.

The Primal Blueprint. 2009. Primal Blueprint Publishing. Mark Sisson.

21-Day Total Body Transformation. 2016. Primal Blueprint Publishing. Mark Sisson.

The Essentials of Sport and Exercise Nutrition, 3rd edition. 2018. Precision Nutrition, Inc. J. Berardi, et al.

American Journal of Clinical Nutrition. 2005; 81: 341-354. **Origins and Evolution of the Western Diet: Health Implications for the 21st Century.** L. Cordain, et al.

Catching Fire: How Cooking Made Us Human. 2010. Basic Books. Richard Wrangham.

American Journal of Clinical Nutrition. 2006 February; 83(2): 211-220. **Effect of a High-Protein Breakfast on the Postprandial Ghrelin Response.** W. Blom, et al.

Nutrition and Metabolism. 2005 September 20; 2: 25. Published online. **Dietary Protein Intake and Renal Function.** William Martin.

Practical Paleo: A Customized Approach to Health and a Whole-Foods Lifestyle. 2012. Victory Belt Publishing. Diane Sanfilippo.

Melatonin. 1996. Bantam Books. Russel Reiter and Jo Robinson.

Scientific Reports. 2017; 7: 11079. **Omega-3 Fatty Acids Correlate with Gut Microbiome Diversity and Production of**

N-carbamylglutamate in Middle Aged and Elderly Women. C. Menni, et al.

Neuroimage. 2016 Jan 15; 125: 988-995. **Magnetic Resonance Spectroscopy Reveals Oral Lactobacillus Promotion of Increases in Brain GABA, N-acetyl Aspartate and Glutamate.** R. Janik, et al.

Biological Psychiatry. 2001 April 1; 49(7): 637-643. **Vagal Modulation of Responses to Mental Challenge in Posttraumatic Stress Disorder.** T. Sahar, et al.

Gut. 2006 October; 55(10): 1512–1520. **Alterations in intestinal permeability.** M. Arrieta, et al.

Neuroscience and Biobehavioral Reviews. 2011 January; 35(3): 565-572. **Sex Bias in Neuroscience and Biomedical Research.** I. Zucker and A.K. Beery.

Women's Voices for the Earth. **15 Toxic Trespassers.** Published online. https://womensvoices.org

Chemical Research in Toxicology. 2014. 27 (5): 834–842. **Progression of Breast Cancer Cells Was Enhanced by Endocrine-Disrupting Chemicals, Triclosan and Octylphenol, Via an Estrogen Receptor-Dependent Signaling Pathway in Cellular and Mouse Xenograft Models.** Hye-Rim Lee, et al.

David Suzuki Foundation. **The Dirty Dozen.** Published online. https://davidsuzuki.org

Andrew Weil, M.D. **How Bad are Artificial Sweeteners?** Published online. https://drweil.com

Outside Online. **Stacy Sims's War on Sports Drinks.** https://outsideonline.com. Aaron Gulley.

https://www.niehs.nih.gov. 2018 November; *National Institute of Environmental Health Sciences.* **High Exposure to Radio Frequency Radiation Associated With Cancer in Male Rats.** News Release.

https://childrenshealthdefense.org. Children's Health Defense. **Too Many Sick Children; Understanding the Basics of Glyphosate; Weeding Out Vaccine Toxins: MMR, Glyphosate, and the Health of a Generation.** Robert F. Kennedy, Jr; Howard Vlieger; Dr. Stephanie Seneff.

www.cdc.gov/vaccines/vac-gen/additives.htm. Centers for Disease Control and Prevention. **What's in Vaccines?**

www.fda.gov/BiologicsBloodVaccines/Vaccines/ApprovedProducts/ucm093833.htm. The Food and Drug Administration. **Vaccine Excipient Summary.**

Cows Save the Planet. 2013. Chelsea Green Publishing. Judith Schwartz.

Gut-Thyroid Connection. Michael Ruscio, D.C. Published online. *https://drruscio.com*

https://www.hrsa.gov/vaccine-compensation/data/index.html. Health Resources and Services Administration. **Vaccine Injury Compensation Data.**

Journal of Sports Science. 2011; 29: S29-38. **Dietary Protein for Athletes: From Requirements to Optimum Adaptation.** S. Phillips and L. Van Loon.

Journal of the American Medical Association. **The Protein-Sparing Action of Carbohydrates.** 2017; (17): 1233

The Hill. 27 June, 2017; **Pediatricians' Group Deeply Alarmed at EPA's Pesticide Decision.** Published online. http://thehill.com. Timothy Cama.

International Archives of Occupational and Environmental Health. 2005; 78(1): 44-50. **Dermal Absorption of Chlorpyrifos in Human Volunteers.** W.A. Meuling, et al.

My Avid Golfer. 2017 August 1; **Golf Course Living: The Good, the Bad, and the Painful.** Published online. https://myavidgolfer.com.

https://beyondpesticides.org. 1995 December; **Toxic Fairways: Risking Groundwater Contamination from Pesticides on Long**

Island Golf Courses. Office of the New York Attorney General, Environmental Protection Bureau.

Meat: A Benign Extravagance. 2010. Chelsea Green Publishing. Simon Fairlie.

Journal of Personality and Social Psychology. 2010 December; 99(6): 1025-1041. **Whatever Does Not Kill Us: Cumulative Lifetime Adversity, Vulnerability, and Resilience.** M. Seery, et al.

http://www.annmariegianni.com. **Ingredient Watch List: Ethanolamines (MEA, DEA, & TEA)—Potential Carcinogens.** 2012.

The Paleo Solution. 2011. Victory Belt Publishing. Robb Wolf.

Journal of the American Medical Association. 2000; 284(4): 483-485. **Is US Health Really the Best in the World?** Barbara Starfield, MD, MPH.

https://www.iarc.fr/wp-content/uploads/2018/07/pr208_E.pdf. International Agency for Research on Cancer. May 31, 2011. **IARC Classifies Radiofrequency Electromagnetic Fields as Possibly Carcinogenic to Humans.** Press Release.

https://ntp.niehs.nih.gov/whatwestudy/topics/cellphones/index.html. National Toxicology Program. November 2018. **Cell Phone Radio Frequency Radiation.**

Consumer Reports. January 27, 2015. Published online. **The Surprising Dangers of CT Scans and X-rays.**

Made in the USA
Monee, IL
05 November 2020